PSYCHING
OUT DIABETES

PSYCHING OUT DIABETES

A Positive Approach to Your Negative Emotions

**Richard R. Rubin, Ph.D.,
June Biermann *and* Barbara Toohey**

LOWELL HOUSE
LOS ANGELES
CONTEMPORARY BOOKS
CHICAGO

LIBRARY OF CONGRESS CATALOGING-IN-PUBLICATION DATA
Rubin, Richard R.
  Psyching out diabetes: A positive approach to your negative emotions / Richard R.
  Rubin and June Biermann and Barbara Toohey.
      p.   cm.
  Includes index.
  ISBN 0-929923-97-9
  1. Diabetes—Psychological aspects.   I. Biermann, June.   II. Toohey, Barbara.
III. Title.
  RC660.R73   1992
  616.4'62—dc20
                                                                    91-44225
                                                                    CIP

The following publishers have generously given permission to use extended quotations
from copyrighted works:

From *Growing Younger,* by Gershon Lesser. Copyright ©1990 by Gershon M. Lesser.
Reprinted with permission from Jeremy P. Tarcher, Inc., Los Angeles, CA.

From *Peace, Love and Healing,* by Bernie Siegel. Copyright ©1989 by Bernard S. Siegel,
M.D. Reprinted by permission of Harper Collins Publishers.

From *Diabetes: Caring for Your Emotions As Well As Your Health,* by J. Edelwich and
A. Brodsky. Copyright ©1986 by Jerry Edelwich and Archie Brodsky. Reprinted with
permission of Addison-Wesley Publishing Company.

Excerpt from an article by Marie Ragghianti reprinted by permission of the author and
the author's agents, Scott Meredith Literary Agency, Inc., 845 Third Avenue, New York,
New York, 10022.

Publisher: Jack Artenstein
Executive Vice President: Nick Clemente
Vice President/Editor-in-Chief: Janice Gallagher
Design: Gary Hespenheide
Manufactured in the United States of America
10 9 8 7 6 5 4 3 2 1

TABLE OF CONTENTS

To Stefan and Mary Sue for the years we've spent psyching out diabetes and for the years to come; to Joseph P. Napora, Ph.D., with whom I developed many of the ideas contained in this book; and to my patients for all they have taught me.

—R. R.

To Ron Hunter with love and admiration for his work for diabetes and his personal integrity and courage.

—J. B. and B. T.

My love affair with June Biermann and Barbara Toohey began shortly after I was diagnosed. My big fear at that time was that I was going to have to give up all the travel that my career demanded, but a friend gave me a copy of *The Peripatetic Diabetic,* which detailed Barbara and June's world travels and I never worried again.

I met Richard Rubin in 1991 at the AADE (American Association of Diabetes Educators) National Convention. We did an interview together about coping with diabetes. His positive outlook, insight, and sense of humor made him an instant friend and ally.

But this foreword is not intended to detail my relationship with the authors. It's to talk about this book and its relationship to diabetes.

Let's face it, diabetes sucks. You not only have to deal with a chronic illness, but with the rest of your life as well. All the other ". . . heartaches and thousand natural shocks that flesh is heir to . . ." do not go away the day you find out you have diabetes.

That's what this book is about—coping—coping with diabetes and coping with life. You cannot separate your diabetes from the rest of your life because everything that affects you will affect your diabetes, just as your diabetes will color everything else in your life. This book will help you integrate diabetes *into* your life, not segregate it *from* your life. What the authors so eloquently point out is that the coping skills you need to deal with diabetes are the very skills you need to deal with day-to-day existence.

The other great thing about this book is that it is written by people who have been there.

My father was diagnosed with Type I diabetes when I was three years old. I grew up watching my parents deal with his disease in the most positive manner imaginable. I never thought of him as being sick, he was just like every other dad except he took two shots a day.

When I was diagnosed with Type I diabetes 32 years later, the news was not as distressing as it might have been. True, I was upset but I had a positive role model and a built-in support group. When I called my parents to tell them, I got more than sympathy—I got empathy.

And empathy is very important. Sympathy will make you feel better in the short run but empathy is what's going to get you through the long haul.

June, Barbara, and Richard are loaded with empathy. They have lived with diabetes. They speak with the knowledge, concern, and tenderness which only those who have lived with it can speak. Reading this book was like a phone call to my mom and dad.

—Tom Parks, *Founder of the American Diabetes Association's Comedy Crusade Against Diabetes*

EMOTIONS: THE FIRST LINE OF DEFENSE

➤ **By June Biermann and Barbara Toohey**

We once attended a dinner party at which the guests included a psychiatrist and his wife. Just as we were sitting down to eat, the phone rang. It was for the psychiatrist. He had given the number to a patient who was going through a particularly difficult time and who might need his help.

As the psychiatrist left the room to answer the phone, his wife merrily shouted after him, "Tell him to pull himself together, Sam."

Over the years, thousands of diabetics have been told, in effect, to pull themselves together and go on about their business. They've usually been told this by people who had no more idea what they were going through than the psychiatrist's wife did. Nor were they given any specific instructions on exactly how to "pull themselves together."

June, now diabetic for 25 years, has somehow managed to keep herself pretty much pulled together. She attributes this to Barbara's loyal support and to the unique opportunity she's had to learn positive thoughts and actions through innumerable conversations with other diabetics we've met through our books and speeches, and through attending many professional conferences over the years. But a certain number of psychoglitches have occurred along the way.

When she was first diagnosed, June sat down to a dismal "last supper" with friends, believing it would be the last time she could ever have a glass of wine, the last time she could ever eat just what she wanted—and as much as she wanted—with never a thought for what the meal might be doing to her blood-sugar level. (In those days little, if any, dietary counseling was available for diabetics.) A few weeks later she spent a long, soul-searching, tearful night trying to figure out how she could face the future alone, having decided that none of her friends would ever want to have anything to do with her because she—and her diabetes—would be such a drag.

A year later she was in Munich attending the Oktoberfest. By then she knew by reading library books on nutritional analysis that she could have a little beer (although certainly not the half-liter they like to serve in Germany!). After having fought taking insulin for nine months, losing so much weight she resembled a Giacometti statue, she finally had accepted the fact that she needed to go "on the needle." As a result, her diabetes was now in fairly decent control. That alone gave her an optimistic feeling that she had lacked before. She had lost no friends and was dining out with relative ease just as in the Before Diabetes days. Yet still, for no logical reason, she spent her last night in Munich weeping and mourning over how wonderful the trip had been and how she might never be able to experience such happiness again. (We now realize this was simply part of the grief response and mourning period that all diabetics pass through.) The waitress in the restaurant where we had dinner overheard June carrying on about how the joy of this perfect trip would soon be over, never to return again, and she didn't raise June's spirits much by telling her, with Teutonic philosophical resignation, "All things must pass."

Fortunately, what eventually passed were June's feelings that life as she knew it and loved it was over because of diabetes. But these feelings surely didn't pass as quickly, as easily, or as painlessly as they could have if she'd had some real understanding of what was going on in her psyche or if she'd had some knowledgeable guidance and counsel along the way.

Oh, Barbara was always there doing her supportive best, telling June, like the psychiatrist's wife, to pull herself together and that everything would be fine. In the same way, your friends and family members are probably doing their supportive best for you; but welcome though it is, this sort of buck-up, optimistic encouragement just doesn't do the job.

We particularly remember one night during an author interview on the Larry King show when we were taking phone calls from the listening audience. A man who had a diabetic wife called in and said that no matter how he tried to help her and no matter how comforting and reassuring he tried to be, she wouldn't take care of her diabetes because she felt, "What's the use? My life is ruined." "What can I do?" he asked helplessly. We rattled on about giving her lots of hugs and showing her unqualified love and kindness and understanding (which he was undoubtedly already doing) and helping her develop her self-esteem so she would want to control her diabetes. We didn't say *how* he could do all of this, because frankly at that time we didn't know how.

Questions like this set us thinking. They brought home to us the fact that for many people, the effect of diabetes on the mind and emotions is its most devastating aspect. In the ensuing years, in letters from reader after reader we were made increasingly aware of their emotional upheavals by comments such as:

"I will not let anyone know I am diabetic."

"I have felt many times that my diabetes is like a gray cloud that always follows over me. I am forever waiting for the rain to come."

"I hate the very word and can hardly say it."

"I am angry about the toll it is taking."

"Friends, family, and co-workers are either of a mind that diabetes is no more serious than a hangnail or they look at you as if you have only 24 hours to live."

These people wrote to us, not because we were experts in psychotherapy, but because they had no one else to turn to and because, as one woman put it, "Life is much easier when you can share your problems with someone who has gone through similar ordeals." Another reason they gave was that we were among the few writers who did not specialize in what they called the gloom-and-doom variety of educational books on diabetes.

Perhaps part of the reason we received so many personal communications was that many doctors and nurses had offered these people little or no help for the frustration of trying to fit diabetes into their lives. One woman wrote us: "Over the 22 years I have lived with diabetes I have never seen a doctor who truly understands what it's like to live with a chronic illness."

Another woman, Joan Hoover—the mother of a diabetic daughter—writing back in 1982 in *Nursing Management of Diabetes Mellitus,* valiantly tried to make health professionals realize that the big barrier to successful treatment was their "inattention to their patient's emotional health." She pointed out that "Most patients are troubled more by the emotional factors associated with diabetes than by its biomedical aspects. However, it is in the emotional area that they are least likely to receive support and guidance. . . . Patients have an intense emotional involvement with their disease. . . . Good diabetes management cannot be achieved without careful and constant monitoring by the patients, themselves. Therefore it is essential that they be in good emotional health to provide that self-care."

Unfortunately, psychological help for diabetics was seldom the first line of defense, but rather a last resort. ("When all else fails, send 'em to a shrink.") For quite a while, we're chagrined to admit, we indulged in this warped thinking ourselves. We recall the times at the SugarFree Center when we did our personal best to help people gain control and accept their diabetes. Then, when nothing else seemed to work, we'd finally, reluctantly say, "Well, I guess there's nothing left for you to do but [discreetly lowering the voice] go for some psychological counseling."

Gradually we changed our attitude. Over the years we saw and heard from more and more people: Type I's (insulin-dependent) and Type II's (non-insulin-dependent), men and women, young and old, newly diagnosed, and long-term residents of the Land of Diabetes—all running through the entire gamut of diabetes-induced emotions of denial, fear, anxiety, anger, guilt, hostility, depression, and frustration. There were some who, like the wife of the caller to Larry King's show, had totally given up on themselves. We wrung our brains to try to come up with something that would bring these people back into the mainstream of a joyful, productive life.

From what readers have told us, we know that our books helped some of them and that June's living example that It Can Be Done helped others. Yet we know the lives of innumerable people with diabetes—and the lives of those who love them—are still being poisoned by a miasma of negative thoughts and emotions.

This shouldn't be. At this point in diabetes history and with the new equipment and therapeutic techniques, it's finally possible for most people to handle the physical problem of diabetes—that is, to maintain close-to-normal blood sugars. More and more scientific evidence points to the fact that good blood-sugar control prevents complications and gives you the freedom and flexibility to lead whatever life you want. Why, then, isn't everyone recognizing this and taking charge of their diabetes and living happily ever after? Why do so many diabetics still experience an all-pervasive discouragement?

In many cases, it's because the mind and body aren't working together in positive harmony; in fact they're engaged in a protracted battle. Never underestimate the power of a negative mind. It can and will drag your body down and keep you from controlling your diabetes and your life.

So you may ask, as the man on Larry King's program did, "What can I do?"

We believe we have at last found some answers for you. Or, rather, we have found a man who has found the answers for you because he has been working on them both professionally and personally for 33 years. His name is Dr. Richard Rubin, and he was delivered unto us when we—and you—needed him most.

In the spring of 1990 we were invited to speak to the Annual Meeting of the Maryland American Diabetes Association Affiliate in Baltimore. As chairman of the board, Dr. Rubin was conducting the meeting. Before and after our talk, we had a chance to get acquainted with him. His credentials were impeccable—Ph.D. in social psychology, Certified Mental Health Counselor, and Certified Diabetes Educator. He was on the staff of the Diabetes Center and Pediatric Diabetes Clinic of

Johns Hopkins Hospital in Baltimore, and he also had a private Diabetes Consultation Service for Counseling and Coping Skills Training. But more important to us, he had a passionate interest in helping diabetics because of two diabetic family members, and he projected a rare combination of strength and gentleness. We discovered that he, too, recognized the need to place emotions right up there in the diabetes hierarchy along with diet, medication, and exercise. On the plane flying back from Baltimore we decided that it was meant to be: we should collaborate with Dr. Rubin on this book. Back home, we immediately got in touch with him and were delighted to discover that he had come to the same logical conclusion. So here we all stand together, ready and eager and able to help you leap over the emotional hurdles of diabetes.

Our goal with this book is to do for you what Emerson said a friend should—to make you be what you can be. At the same time we want to emulate Civil War General George McClellan, who, when Lincoln returned him to his battered and discouraged troops, rode among them infusing them with enthusiasm, strength, and hope.

➤ **By Richard R. Rubin, Ph.D.**

My life with diabetes began 33 years ago, in 1959, when my sister was diagnosed. I was 16 and she was 9. We're very close, so like anybody who loves someone with diabetes, I lived with it even though I didn't have it.

I remember life with diabetes back then: staggering into the bathroom first thing in the morning to urinate and seeing my sister's syringe sterilizer boiling away on the back of the toilet tank, watching her sharpen her needles with steel wool (in the days before anyone dreamed of disposable syringes), looking on as she read her urine sugar results from the Clinitest tablets and neatly entered them in her log book. Most of all, though, I remember not talking about her diabetes. None of us did. My family tended to take a stiff-upper-lip approach to all misfortunes, and that was the way we dealt with Mary Sue's diabetes. My parents seemed to believe that talking about problems only made them worse. Looking back, I realize that the silence made me feel that diabetes was too awful to talk about.

This feeling was reinforced by an experience I had the year after my sister's diagnosis. For some reason, everyone in the eleventh grade was given urine tests for diabetes. All the boys in my class trooped over to the locker room, all except one who stayed behind. When we returned from the test I asked my classmate why he hadn't joined us. He stared at me for a moment, then blurted out tearfully, "I've got a disease."

The message was clear: Diabetes was too terrible to discuss. Images of amputations, blindness, horrible embarrassing insulin reactions. Hush, hush. Don't talk or you might wake the bogeyman.

Fast-forward almost exactly 20 years. I can still remember the date—April 4, 1979—I sat with my seven-year-old son and my wife in our pediatrician's office, confirming what we had feared: Stefan had diabetes. His symptoms over the past two weeks had been unmistakable: unquenchable thirst and waking up many times each night to urinate. Our pediatrician, Doctor Bill, was an old friend from my college days. As he gently listed all the requirements and restrictions that would guide us as we began our journey with diabetes, I felt like screaming, "No! It can't be true! I can't deal with this!"

Actually, after the initial shock of Stefan's diagnosis, the next few months were relatively easy. We basked in the glow of his diabetes "honeymoon"—that period immediately after diagnosis of Type I diabetes when insulin therapy begins and the diabetes goes into remission, a period that invariably gives parents the false hope that their child doesn't really have diabetes after all.

Day after day Stefan's Clinitest tablets turned that reassuring beautiful deep blue color that signified a negative urine sugar. He had no reaction, no problems with his new diet or with his single low-dosage (only 2 units) shot of insulin a day. Just like every other parent before me I couldn't resist the thought that maybe the diagnosis was wrong; maybe he didn't have diabetes. And even if he did, handling it was (you should pardon the expression) a piece of cake.

Like all honeymoons, ours came to an end all too soon. Suddenly, after about six months, the Clinitest results were no longer blue, but various earth tones of green, orange, and muddy brown, which I quickly learned to hate because they indicated high sugar content in the urine and out-of-control diabetes. The truth was that we had been granted a brief respite after Stefan's diagnosis, as his pancreas waged its final, futile battle to keep producing insulin. Now it was time to get on with our real life with diabetes.

Real life with diabetes was complicated. We measured and balanced and adjusted and worried. Our former footloose lifestyle was a thing of the past. Preparing to leave the house was a throwback to our days with babies, only instead of diapers, bottles, and extra clothes, we had to lug testing supplies, snacks, and insulin. Sometimes Stefan's control was bad, no matter how hard we worked to get it right. Often we felt that our entire lives revolved around managing his diabetes. When things weren't going well, Stefan would get frustrated or guilty, scared or resentful, and so would I. My parents and sister had lived with these same feelings two decades before, and I was determined to deal with them differently.

At about this time I read an article with a title something like "Good metabolic control; Is it attainable? Is it desirable?" It got me thinking about the whole issue of balance as the key to living well with diabetes. Everyone was telling us about balance, but the message was limited to issues of balancing food, exercise, and insulin. Somehow, I sensed that leaving feelings out of the equation made a true balance impossible. It seemed that we had to learn to work with our feelings, just as we worked with the other elements of the regimen. We had to learn to psych out diabetes, because the only alternative was to let it psych us out.

So my career in psyching out diabetes was launched. At first my motivation was strictly personal. I wanted Stefan to grow up emotionally strong as well as physically healthy, and I wanted to maintain the wonderful, relaxed, confident life my family had led before he developed diabetes. I read everything I could find that might help me. Unfortunately, it was precious little. I also talked to many other people who were living with diabetes, and I found enlightenment and comfort in these conversations.

After a few years I felt I had learned enough about the art and science of psyching out diabetes to begin sharing what I knew in my clinical practice as a mental-health counselor. Over the past decade I have worked with thousands of people who live with diabetes—in my offices, in hospital clinics, at lectures I've given, and in various research studies. Everywhere I go I'm on the lookout for new lessons, new tricks that work to psych out diabetes, and I'm amazed how often I find them. The people with whom I work are my teachers, and I hope they will be yours, through the stories I will tell you in this book.

The teachers closest to my heart are my first ones, my sister Mary Sue and my son Stefan. Today Mary Sue is in good shape physically, considering the fact that she has had diabetes for 33 years and much of that time was before today's more effective therapies were developed. Mary Sue is in good shape emotionally, as well. In her own special way, she has learned to psych out diabetes.

Stefan has, too. He's 20 now, and we've both somehow survived his teenage years. Like most young people, he often feels the need to do things his way rather than by the book, and I respect and love him for his independence. He's managed to maintain remarkably good metabolic control, by means I frequently find unfathomable.

Speaking of psyching out diabetes brings to mind two of the most dedicated psycher-outers of all, my coauthors, June Biermann and Barbara Toohey. June and Barbara have been heroines of mine for years. They have written some of the wisest and most inspiring books ever written about diabetes and, in the course of their work, have evolved some unique diabetes therapies, including my personal favorite: hug therapy.

Imagine my delight when, two years ago, I learned that they had been invited to give the keynote speech at the annual meeting of my state American Diabetes Association affiliate. I used my position as affiliate chairman of the board to wangle the honor of introducing them to the audience. I concluded my remarks by confessing a long-held secret wish—that I would someday meet June and Barbara in person, and that each of them would give me a great big hug. They did. Not long after, we decided to write this book, which I hope you enjoy reading as much as I enjoyed writing.

Please read the following preliminary information: 1) For Diabetics and 2) Help for Those Who Want to Help Diabetics.

➤ For Diabetics

In this book we will first discuss what we've all come to think of as the "bad" emotions: denial, obsession, anger, depression, and so on. But nothing is all bad. These feelings may be painful to experience, but like physical pain, they serve a useful purpose. Without physical pain you would hold onto a hot pan until your flesh charred. You would walk around with a rock in your shoe until you ground a hole in your foot. Without the symptomatic pain of a headache or stomachache, you would let a serious but correctable problem go on until it was too late. It has been said that pain is our friend because it alerts us that something is wrong so that we can fix it.

The same can be said of emotional pain. The negative emotions are what Dr. Rubin calls smoke alarms. They wake you up so you can get yourself out of danger.

Everyone is susceptible to negative emotions. They are part of the human condition. But when you have diabetes and it comes to negative emotions, it seems that you're more human than anybody. Whether you're newly diagnosed or have had diabetes for a number of years, you find panic, fear, anger, guilt, shame, depression, and grief raising their ugly heads more often than you remember them doing in your prediabetic days and certainly, it seems, more often with you than with your nondiabetic friends.

You're probably right. After all, you have a built-in reason for feeling bad. You have a chronic disease, one that imposes restrictions and routines on your life, one that, if you don't toe the line of care and control, may lead to complications, and one that in itself can upset your hormonal balance and give you regular rides on an emotional roller coaster.

You're also probably wrong. Many of the negative emotions you're experiencing have nothing to do with your diabetes, but since diabetes makes such a handy scapegoat, it's only natural to load all your emotional problems onto its head. You think that if it weren't for this rotten disease, your life would be a barrel of monkeys. Even many of the negative emotions you experience that actually do have something to do with your diabetes are often a result not of the disease itself but of your lack of knowledge of the skills that will keep it from changing your mood and messing up your emotions.

Emotions are something like blood sugar. As a diabetic your blood sugar levels may be crazy for no reason that you can think of. You've eaten the right foods, done your normal amount of exercise, haven't been under any unusual stress, and yet here you are with a 275 blood sugar—or a 48. What do you do? Well, what you shouldn't do is anguish, fret, and rant and mutter that diabetes is impossible. You shouldn't throw up your hands in despair and go eat a hot fudge sundae because nothing works anyway. No, you should fix it. If your blood sugar is low, take your glucose tablet or Lifesavers or Coke or whatever and raise it. If it's high, take a little corrective insulin or a little less food and a little more exercise (or both) and bring it down.

It's the same with your emotions. When you plunge into an emotional Grand Canyon, don't just figure that the Demon Diabetes pushed you and that no matter what you do you're not going to get out, that you're stuck down there until the buzzards come to pick your bones. Don't just label diabetes hopeless and yourself helpless and give up and go eat a hot fudge sundae because nothing works anyway. No, do something to fix it. Get rid of those negative emotions!

Now, admittedly it's harder and takes longer to get rid of powerful negative emotions than to correct a low or high blood sugar, but still it can be done. There are techniques you can learn and destructive emotional habits you can unlearn, and Dr. Rubin will show you how. It will take some time and effort on your part, but you'll find it's well worth it. Then not only will you have a more realistic and optimistic attitude toward your diabetes, but toward your life as well. You won't just climb out of the emotional Grand Canyon onto the flatland; you'll have earned a chance—at least occasionally— to experience the beautiful emotions, to scale an emotional Everest where you'll breathe the rarefied atmosphere of exultant joy. So strap on your crampons, pick up your climbing rope and ice axe, and let us begin.

➤ Help for Those Who Want to Help Diabetics

If you want to give the diabetic person in your life a boost over the psychological hurdles associated with diabetes, you should read all of the material in this book for background to help you gain an understanding of what the person is going through.

But we realize that diabetes causes you to have problems, too. For that reason, at the end of each chapter (except the last one) we have a section especially for you. The information there will help you cope with the unique problems you face as you try to help your diabetic loved one cope with the problems he or she faces.

PSYCHING
OUT DIABETES

DENIAL
WHICH NOBODY CAN DENY

Let us take you on a little adventure in Jargonland. Now hear this: "The basic problem is that he/she is still in *denial.*" "I just don't know what to do to get some *compliance* out of him/her." "At this rate he/she is never going to be *empowered.*" These phrases and variations thereon are often used by health professionals, and they're talking about you. What do they mean? Basically, they mean you aren't taking care of your diabetes. When they say you're in denial, they mean that even if you've been diagnosed for years, even if you take insulin or pills, even if your diabetes has landed you in the hospital a few times, even if you wear a diabetes ID bracelet, deep down inside in your heart of hearts and soul of souls you still don't admit to the fact that you have diabetes. That being the case, it stands to reason that you won't be compliant—in other words, you won't do all those things they're telling you (for your own good) you should be doing to keep the diabetes (that you don't really admit you have) in control. Therefore, it is extremely unlikely that they'll be able to empower you, meaning get you to take charge of your diabetes and assume responsibility for your own care.

While complaining about how health professionals fling around such jargon we have to admit that these people have a tough row to hoe. When dealing with you they have to walk a psychological line as narrow as the line you walk between high and low blood sugar. Let's say they tell you, as one newly diagnosed college student said she was told by the head nurse, "You have a dreadful, dreadful disease." This convinced her that all she had to look forward to in life was "becoming a blind, bilateral amputee, carried off to dialysis three times a week."

If you're told something like this, it stands to reason that you may be so shocked and frightened at the thought of facing such a horrible future that you deny you have diabetes ("This has nothing to do with me!") and consequently don't do what you need to do to keep your diabetes in control and prevent these dire predictions from coming true.

On the other hand, health professionals who are overly concerned about not frightening you may soft-pedal the diagnosis and the consequences of neglect. They may tell you something like, "You just have borderline diabetes" (there's no such animal), or "Diabetes is no big deal. You just have to avoid sugar and take these pills (or a little insulin) and you'll be fine. You can lead a perfectly normal life. Don't worry." Since you're more than willing to consider it no big deal and not to worry about it, you just shrug off your diabetes and don't bother doing what you need to do to keep the disease in control and keep it from becoming a big deal.

Organizations soliciting funds for diabetes research have to walk this same narrow line. If their ads and radio and TV announcements don't make diabetes sound like the greatest scourge to hit the planet since the black plague, people aren't going to be inspired to open their purses to contribute to find a cure. On the other hand, if they paint diabetes in colors of unmitigated horror, diabetics and their families are going to get scared into deep denial.

We've talked a lot about denial here, but you may still be a little uncertain as to what it actually is. You may be like the man who went on a safari to shoot (photographically speaking, of course) elephants. The problem was he hadn't a clue as to what an elephant looked like. When he came back to the camp at the end of the day, everybody asked him how his expedition had gone. "Bad luck!" he said. "I didn't see a single elephant anywhere. Actually there wasn't even room for an elephant out there because the place was so full of huge gray animals with long, funny snouts and big, fanlike ears and ropy tails."

In this chapter, we're going to ask Dr. Rubin to show you exactly what the elephant of denial looks like and how it behaves so you can recognize it and—if you find you have it—send it packing back to the dark continent where it belongs.

—June and Barbara

June and Barbara: Let's begin at the beginning: the diagnosis. When unmistakable symptoms indicate and medical tests confirm that a person has diabetes, is it common to deny the diagnosis itself? We ask this because we were amazed that both of the endocrinologists who coauthored books with us, Lois Jovanovic-Peterson (*The Diabetic Woman*) and Peter Lodewick (*The Diabetic Man*), were totally unable to accept their own diagnoses.

This is how Lois described her situation:

> I had completed medical school and was in the middle of my endocrine/metabolism fellowship when it happened to me. I completely denied the symptoms. I attributed my weight loss, irritability, and insomnia (which was caused by my constant need to urinate during the night) to the stress of my career.
>
> Then, during the middle of an experiment, I donated my blood as a normal control. When it came back sky-high— more than three times the normal range—I thought the assay was wrong. When my blood was used to calibrate the biostater (a kind of giant mechanical pancreas used in hospitals), I did not think that the 400 blood sugar might be mine, but instead screamed at the technician that she was not calibrating the machine correctly.
>
> After three months of deteriorating health, I was forced by a dear friend and colleague to admit the truth.

Pete's story is similar:

> I'd just completed the grueling years of medical school
> and medical internship and was contemplating reaping
> the benefits of all the hard labor I had put into my
> lifelong dream of becoming a doctor when the symptoms
> of diabetes struck.
>
> As I reflect on it, I'm sure that consciously or
> unconsciously I felt that diabetes was an attack on me
> as a man. Before I could even accept the *possibility* that
> I had diabetes, I rationalized a lot. Even my typical
> symptoms of high blood sugar—extreme thirst, excessive
> urination—getting up several times in the night for trips
> to the bathroom—fatigue and weight loss—couldn't
> convince me that I was diabetic. I foolishly ignored these
> symptoms.
>
> After several months of intense symptoms of high
> blood sugar, my six-foot-three-inch frame had dwindled
> to 152 pounds. As a doctor, I was being that much more
> of a fool to continue to deny diabetes any longer.

If knowledgeable professionals can blind themselves to
strong factual evidence in this manner, what chance does the
ordinary person have to face up to the diagnosis and not allow
the mind to block out the truth?

Dr. Rubin: Both Dr. Jovanovic-Peterson and Dr. Lodewick
have Type I (insulin-dependent) diabetes. In my experience,
denying the diagnosis of Type I diabetes is rare. Given the
dramatic symptoms that accompany the onset of Type I diabetes, very few people deny as long or as vehemently as Pete
and Lois did. I'd guess that both of them were strongly predisposed by their personalities (and perhaps by their professional roles as well) to fight tooth and nail the notion that they
could be laid low by a chronic disease in the prime of life and
at the launching of their medical careers. In medical school
during the years when they were diagnosed, the curriculum

may have been weighted more heavily toward chronicling the complications of diabetes than toward describing the new techniques of control that could prevent those complications.

I do know one woman who denied her Type I diabetes despite dramatic symptoms, but she did this for a distinctive reason. When she started losing weight, she held off going to the doctor to see what was wrong because it was such a pleasure for her to lose weight so effortlessly. Finally, after she had lost about 30 pounds and was at what she considered her ideal weight, she saw a doctor and received the diagnosis.

June and Barbara: Another diabetic woman, also Type I, told us a somewhat similar story. When she had undiagnosed diabetes she started shedding pounds, as the woman above did, and on top of that, diabetes caused her face to be flushed an attractive, rosy color. Everyone told her how wonderful she looked—Glowing! Absolutely fabulous! Then, because of the development of other less flattering symptoms, she went to the doctor and discovered the source of her new allure: diabetes.

Fortunately this woman is a scientist and professor of microbiology and she well knew how fleeting this beauty would be—and how permanent the complications would be—if she didn't get her diabetes in control, so she set about doing that immediately. She did not for a moment try to deny her diabetes for cosmetic reasons.

If Type I's with their vivid symptoms can sometimes manage to deny diabetes, it must be a cinch for those with the subtle, almost unnoticeable symptoms of Type II diabetes (non–insulin-dependent) to pretend to themselves they are not diabetic even after diagnosis.

Dr. Rubin: Yes, it's much more common, and this denial can go on for years and be very destructive. The reason, of course, is that the symptoms are so much less dramatic that it's extremely easy to ignore them. With Type II's there's an interesting parallel to Peter and Lois's denial of their Type I diabetes: people who should know better are often world-class deniers.

I know a social worker who spends his working life helping people deal with their problems, yet his denial of his Type II diabetes is so strong that he can't even remember how long he's had it. One woman has seen her mother and five sisters die because they refused to care for their diabetes—yet she's following in their footsteps right to the grave.

June and Barbara: We've talked with a number of Type II diabetics whose doctors minimized the importance of the diagnosis so much that the patients got the impression it was something they could dismiss for the time being. You might call this a form of doctor-induced denial. Have you had experience with people who use their doctor's soft-pedaling of the diagnosis as an excuse for not really accepting diabetes?

Dr. Rubin: Absolutely. Some doctors take a protective attitude and tell patients they have "borderline diabetes" or "just a touch of sugar." One woman who received such a diagnosis told me years later that she decided "borderline" meant no serious problem, and she threw the diet guide she had been given into a drawer. When people tell me they've "only got a touch of sugar," I explain that a touch of sugar is like being a little pregnant. It doesn't describe a real condition. You are either pregnant or you're not; you either have diabetes—and need to deal with it—or you don't.

June and Barbara: The other day we were talking to Rick, a man in his early thirties who has had diabetes for about ten years and now is permanently afflicted with extremely painful neuropathy. He's very resentful that the physician who initially diagnosed his diabetes told him, "Well, you'll probably be all right for about five years, but if you don't change your life [he was drinking, smoking, carousing, subjecting himself to extreme stress in both work and play] you'll be in for trouble—and that means complications."

"You know what that tells a guy in his twenties," said Rick. "It tells him, 'Go ahead and raise hell for another five years. You can worry about your diabetes later.'" And that's just what Rick's doing now: worrying about his diabetes—a lot.

Dr. Rubin: On the other hand, if a doctor uses naked scare tactics, that makes some diabetics feel so hopeless that they refuse to face up to their disease. There's also a third way doctors can create denial in their patients—by taking a "doctor knows best" approach that leaves the diabetic passive and unskilled.

June and Barbara: Why do you think doctors behave in these denial-inducing ways when diagnosing diabetics?

Dr. Rubin: As you mentioned earlier, it's not easy to walk the narrow line between instilling serious concern in the patient and giving comfort and reassurance. Some patients respond better to one approach than the other, and you can't always know ahead of time which way will work with an individual. It's also hard for a doctor to ascertain exactly how much responsibility for the care of the disease a patient can handle, especially in the early stages.

There are also other, less valid, reasons why doctors' actions are sometimes counterproductive in diagnosing diabetics. Some doctors are just not up-to-date with state-of-the-art diabetes care. They may not even recommend home blood-sugar testing, glycohemoglobin testing (a test that tells how overall control has been over the last three months), or more than one insulin shot a day, because they do not know about these more modern and better methods of control.

Other doctors lack skills in providing adequate information to their patients. Some doctors don't take time to answer questions and lack staff trained to teach diabetes self-management. Some have little confidence in the capacities of their patients to learn good self-care. This, combined with their desire to maintain control of the therapeutic process, may cause these doctors to make recommendations like, "I'll test your blood as often as you need it. Just come to my office once a month."

Not all of the blame should be placed on the doctor. As always, it takes two to tango. When you play the part of the passive patient in reaction to any of these approaches by your doctor, you're really letting yourself down. I know it can be hard, but you need to take full responsibility for your personal program of diabetes control. The key here is not what your doctor does, it's what you do. You must become as fully informed as you can about diabetes. Read, go to meetings, talk to other people with the disease. See if they're using techniques that might be good for you. How does their relationship with their doctor compare with yours? Are you satisfied with the way your doctor responds when you tell him or her about things you've learned?

Be assertive with your doctor. You're the one who's going to suffer if you're passive. Before your appointment, write down any questions you want to ask, and state at the beginning of the appointment that you want the doctor to take time to answer them. If you want to discuss some change in your regime, make this clear. Be sure you understand and feel comfortable with your doctor's responses. If you feel you need some special service that has not been offered (nutritional, educational, or psychological counseling, for instance), ask the doctor to provide it or to refer you to someone who can.

As a last resort, be prepared to change doctors. I'd recommend this only if you can't work out a cooperative, constructive relationship with your current physician. Don't give up without making an honest effort. If you must switch, make sure that your new doctor is flexible and willing to listen and learn right along with you. The better informed you are, the more self-management skills you master, the more assertive you are, the less likely you are to deny your diabetes.

June and Barbara: We've seen many people who are actually in double denial—not only denying that they have diabetes, but denying that they're denying. After all, as they logically point out, they *are* taking whatever insulin or medications are required, and they *do* go to the doctor, and they always put down "diabetes" on any form that asks for medical history. You would have a hard time convincing them that even though they're doing all of this, they're still in denial.

Dr. Rubin: First of all, denial rarely means totally blocking out diabetes. Most often denial is the psychological equivalent of the old semipermeable membrane we learned about in high school biology. It lets some of the reality through, but not all. Unfortunately, for many people precious little diabetic reality gets through. Folks may go for years denying the need for any self-care beyond taking their pills or their morning insulin shot. Others don't "get" the relationship between their diet and their weight, or between their weight and their blood sugars. Others never make the connection between symptoms like chronic exhaustion, never-ending infection, or painful neuropathy, and out-of-control diabetes.

June and Barbara: If some diabetics honestly aren't sure whether they're in denial, how can you help them find out?

Dr. Rubin: It's true that recognizing that you're in denial is almost a contradiction in terms. For those who are game and want to do a little self-analysis, I can list some signs of denial. You might check to see if you have any of these signs. If you find you do, you might then gently question yourself about what these signs really mean to you.

1. Do you have symptoms you can't explain, like frequent urination, chronic exhaustion or infections, pains in the arms or legs, or blurry vision?

2. Do you avoid medical care for your diabetes?

3. Do you feel uncomfortable acknowledging that you have diabetes or reading about the disease? (Did you decide to read this book yourself or did someone give it

to you and suggest you read it? Do you already feel like throwing it down and going off to do something else?)

4. Do you tell yourself that you can effectively treat your disease simply by taking pills or insulin shots?

5. Do you ever say that you have "borderline diabetes," or "just a touch of sugar"?

This quiz is something like those you find in magazines and newspapers to see if you're an alcoholic: if you answer yes to any of the questions, it's a good indication you are in denial— that you have a touch of the ostrich syndrome.

June and Barbara: We all know what that means—burying your head in the sand when you feel you're in danger, thinking that if you can't see what's threatening you, you're safe. What would make people do such a bird-brained thing?

Dr. Rubin: On the surface, ostrichlike behavior looks absolutely irrational. Here's this being with his head in the sand, totally ignoring some potentially catastrophic reality. But let's look at it from the ostrich's point of view. From his perspective, he's making the best of a bad situation. If he can't escape physically from whatever fate may befall him, at least he can avoid facing it directly and making his agony even more acute. Some diabetics engage in this very same behavior, for the very same reason.

June and Barbara: And, we would imagine, with the very same results. An ostrich with his head stuck in the sand makes himself totally vulnerable to the fearsome thing he can't bear to face. Diabetics with the ostrich syndrome—never going to the doctor because he or she might tell you something you're afraid to hear, never testing your blood sugar because you know it's going to be high and you can't stand looking at the numbers, and never reading books about diabetes because they scare you with descriptions of potential problems—make themselves vulnerable to the very complications they can't bear to admit they might develop.

Dr. Rubin: That's right. Only there's one big difference between real ostriches and diabetic ostriches: the diabetic variety actually have much more control over their physical fate, they just don't recognize it because their heads are stuck in the sand. They believe they have no power to control their fate, but they do. Even though the fate that diabetics fear is absolutely not inevitable, operating like an ostrich is guaranteed to make it so. It's the classic case of a self-fulfilling prophecy. This works in all areas of life. For example, if I have the dream of someday running a marathon but convince myself I never will, my conviction will keep me from the intensive training I need to make my dream a reality.

June and Barbara: What turns an otherwise rational person into an ostrich? We, personally, have devoted the last 25 years to writing, ranting and raving, demonstrating, and documenting that complications *can* be avoided with good diabetes care, that with the latest diabetes therapies you *can* live a happy, healthy, productive, exciting, rich, full, wonderful life as a diabetic. We know that you and other respected diabetes health professionals have been doing the same thing for your patients with all your hearts and souls and minds. Why won't people hear the good news and act on it?

Dr. Rubin: That's the proverbial $64,000 question. Why would people persist in believing that they can't control their fate when really they can? Beliefs are strange things. They are very powerful. Our behavior, ostrichlike and otherwise, is determined by our beliefs. Some beliefs are buried so deeply in the furthest reaches of our consciousness that they control our behavior almost automatically. These deeply rooted beliefs send us thought messages, to which we react as we might to subliminal messages flashed on the screen at a movie theater directing us to the concession stand.

June and Barbara: How can we tell if our diabetic lives are flying on this kind of automatic-belief pilot?

Dr. Rubin: The only way to tell is by observing your own behavior. You must be able to stop, look at your behavior, and ask yourself, without judgment or defensiveness, whether what you are doing makes sense. Sometimes the answer will be yes. If so, fine. Other times the answer will be no. Ostrich-like behavior regarding diabetes will almost always generate a resounding no, if and when you can approach it in this gentle, straightforward way.

June and Barbara: Okay, let's say we examine what we're doing and acknowledge that it doesn't make sense. Does that make this senseless, ostrichlike behavior magically disappear?

Dr. Rubin: Unfortunately, it's usually not that easy. Up until now you've been operating as if this behavior did make sense, so you can't just suddenly dismiss the thoughts that brought it about and go on your way. You have to disarm these thoughts, and to do that, we have to really get to know them. This part can actually be fun—almost a kind of detective work.

June and Barbara: How about giving us an example? Here's a common situation: a person who refuses to test his blood sugar. Assuming that it's not just a matter of having an aversion to sticking his finger to get the blood, what thoughts and beliefs would lead to this kind of behavior, when the person knows that he has to test his blood frequently in order to know where he stands so he can keep diabetes in control?

Dr. Rubin: The process involved with finding this out reminds me of when I was nine years old, lying in bed with my little crystal radio, delicately twisting the tuning knob, trying to discover a new station. That's what we have to do now: see what thoughts we can tune in. Here are some thoughts my patients have come up with when we discussed this tuning-in process on the subject of testing blood sugars:

> ➤ "My blood sugars are always high, so why even bother testing?"
> ➤ "It's so inconvenient and I just don't have time. I'm simply too busy."
> ➤ "I don't test regularly, so there's really no sense testing at all."
> ➤ "No one else has to do this, why should I?"
> ➤ "My husband [or wife, mother, doctor, or whoever] uses my blood-sugar results as evidence against me. Why should I give them any ammunition?"

June and Barbara: These certainly sound familiar. No doubt individual diabetics will express many more thoughts on the same subject. What produces these thoughts? They don't just come out of nowhere, do they?

Dr. Rubin: No, they come from our beliefs, which—to continue the radio analogy—are like the transmitter-controller for the whole network.

June and Barbara: What kind of beliefs would produce such thoughts?

Dr. Rubin: They could include something like:

> ➤ "I'll never have decent blood sugars. I'll always be out of control no matter what I do."
> ➤ "It's impossible to fit blood-sugar testing into my lifestyle."
> ➤ "I can't stand being different."
> ➤ "It's never safe to be open about your diabetes, even (or especially) with family members and doctors."

June and Barbara: We're beginning to get the idea, but let's have some more examples. What would be the thoughts and underlying beliefs of people who refuse to go to the doctor?

Dr. Rubin: The thoughts might be:

  ➤ "The doctor is not supportive or understanding; always critical or disappointed in me."
  ➤ "Why bother going? The doctor always tells me the same thing, and then I go home and don't do anything I was told to do."
  ➤ "The doctor is always so rushed. It's just in and out. I never have time to ask questions. What's the point?"

The underlying beliefs that produce these thoughts might include:

  ➤ "Doctors are no help at all. I never get any support or suggestions. The only thing I get out of the visit is a bill."
  ➤ "Every time I go to the doctor I feel worse. I get so guilty, depressed, and hopeless. There's no benefit at all."

June and Barbara: Let's do one more—one that particularly hits home with us. What are the thoughts and beliefs of people who refuse to read books about diabetes or go to meetings for diabetics?

Dr. Rubin: A couple of possible thoughts might be:

  ➤ "When I read books about other diabetics, or talk to them, they always make it sound so easy that it makes me feel incompetent or just plain stupid, because it's not that easy for me."
  ➤ "When I read books about diabetes or attend meetings they make diabetes sound so dismally horrible that afterward I feel worse than ever."

Underlying these thoughts could be the belief that:

> ➤ "Information about diabetes only hurts me, making me feel hopeless or inadequate."

June and Barbara: In your experience with patients, how does this tuning-in process affect them?

Dr. Rubin: They usually find several interesting things about it:

1. The process itself isn't hard, as long as it is undertaken in the right spirit—one of gentle, nonjudgmental self-discovery.

2. The thoughts and beliefs uncovered have a paradoxical quality. They are both very familiar and altogether new. That's because you've lived with them for a long time but you've probably never really looked at them closely before.

3. *If*—and this is a very big if—the underlying beliefs that drive the system were true, your ostrichlike behavior would make perfect sense. If you could never control your blood sugars no matter what you did, if there was no benefit to doctor appointments, and if reading about diabetes only hurt you, burying your head in the sand would be totally rational.

June and Barbara: While these underlying beliefs may have a little truth in them, they aren't totally true, are they?

Dr. Rubin: That's just the point. They can't be true because they're absolute. The only absolutes are death and taxes. Nothing about diabetes is absolute. If it seems as though I'm making too big a deal about absoluteness, stop and think a minute. You know you don't really believe that it's literally impossible to control your blood sugars. Extremely difficult? Yes. But impossible? Absolutely not! And there's all the difference in the world between impossible and extremely difficult.

Absolutely negative beliefs lead inevitably to ostrichlike behavior. Anything less than absolute negativity has to lead in other directions. For example, if there is literally no benefit in seeing your doctor, you're wise not to go. If, on the other hand, you are simply dissatisfied with your appointments, myriad possibilities arise for changing the situation. A shift away from absoluteness of even a single degree leads almost inexorably away from head-burying.

June and Barbara: So you have to replace your absolutely negative beliefs with more realistic ones, ones with a glimmer of positiveness and hope, and that will get you out of denial. Is it really that simple?

Dr. Rubin: Yes, it's that simple, but it's not easy. Old beliefs die hard because they're so deeply ingrained. It takes patience, practice, and persistence to accomplish this shift to more realistic beliefs. But it's true that the longest journey begins with a single step.

June and Barbara: To show how this is done, why not walk us through the first steps into more realistic thoughts and beliefs in, for example, controlling blood sugar.

Dr. Rubin: At the most fundamental level, let's say your thoughts are: "I have a really hard time controlling my blood sugar. I hate to see the tests when they're high. It's painful, infuriating, and depressing to test three or four times a day and get awful numbers most of the time, especially when I write them down and see weeks of 200s and 300s staring me in the face every time I open my log book. I know I should test, but I can't unless I can find a way to make it less horrible for me."

This is a start. You've acknowledged what a drag testing is, but you've done this without resorting to absolutes. In the process you've identified your real goal: testing without feeling overwhelmed and depressed. Now you can start brainstorming for ways you might take a first step toward your goal, something like: "I could start by testing just one time a day, maybe even at a time I think I'll get a good number, just to get going. I won't even write down the results at first. If I just start off really easy, my confidence might build."

As soon as you've convinced yourself that it's possible to lift your head out of the sand, you're on the way to putting your ostrich days behind you. Even the tiniest positive action based on realistic beliefs about your diabetes can help you get the sand out of your eyes.

June and Barbara: This all sounds very logical and very possible, but how do you get diabetics in denial to take that first positive action? Small though the step may be, it could look like a giant leap to them.

Dr. Rubin: Your question is posed as if someone else could make diabetics emerge from denial and begin their journey along the paths of diabetic righteousness. Here's a point I'll keep making throughout this book (probably ad nauseam): No one can make anyone else do anything. I prefer to address the question from the point of view of the diabetic, rather than commenting on the impossibility of facilitating change in another person.

June and Barbara: Okay, we get the point. No one else can make you do something or do it for you. How, then, do you get yourself to take those first steps out of denial?

Dr. Rubin: First, you have to keep in mind what puts you into denial in the first place. When you deny, you're trying to transform a painful reality into something less overwhelming. You'll continue to deny as long as the denial costs you less emotionally than facing reality does. You will begin to emerge from denial if this balance shifts, if the benefits of facing reality outweigh those of maintaining your denial.

June and Barbara: It's true that making changes in our lives takes such effort and is often so painful and frightening that it takes something pretty dramatic to nudge us into action. What dramatic somethings have you observed that have triggered that emotional balance shift?

Dr. Rubin: First, something really positive might happen, building your motivation to face reality. Some examples I've heard include falling in love, wanting to have a baby, becoming a grandparent, meeting someone else with diabetes who has a really good attitude, or finding a truly wise and empathetic health-care provider.

June and Barbara: We've certainly seen positive motivations like this in action—particularly wanting to have a baby, a perfect baby. This desire has converted the most self-destructive deniers into paragons of diabetes control and even into evangelists on the subject who want to convert the whole world of diabetics, bless them. But, unfortunately, in our experience negative motivations far outnumber positive ones. It seems that it takes that first harbinger of complications to make a person into a true believer that he or she really does have diabetes. No more denial is possible; changes *must* be made. We're only happy when the complications are caught early enough to be reversed.

Dr. Rubin: Yes, sad to say, the most common reason for emerging from denial is some diabetes-related medical crisis. The examples of this from my practice are innumerable:

➤ After years of ignoring her diabetes, a woman finally becomes so hyperglycemic that she ends up in the hospital and has to go on insulin.

➤ After 20 years of "doing anything he wanted," a man loses an eye to diabetic eye disease. "That really got my attention," he comments.

➤ A woman who lived for 23 years with "mild sugar" develops serious circulation problems, prompting her to observe, "I know now what I should have known all along—that mild sugar means diabetes."

➤ A man who dealt with his diabetes for years by taking his pills, eating what he wanted, and going on his merry way, says, "Now I've got complications, and my way doesn't seem all that merry."

Since most people emerge from denial as a result of something that happens to them, it's hard to offer any tried-and-true guidelines for creating denial-ending motivations. I can't suggest that you precipitate a medical emergency or that you fall in love. (Although on second thought the latter is not a bad idea, if you're not in love already.) That's what makes denial such a tough nut to crack. On the other hand, I'm not suggesting that you are powerless here, that if you're in denial you have to sit around waiting for fate or fortune to strike. You can't get off the responsibility hook that easily.

June and Barbara: One thing we would advise is learning from the mistakes of others. To cite a nondiabetes example of this, a friend of ours was once held at knifepoint for four hours by an intruder who climbed through her bathroom window. When the police arrived to investigate, they said to her, "Jeez, lady, what did you expect? Your bathroom window was open." (Of course it was open—the day had been hot and she was trying to cool off the house.) "And you don't even have any bars on the window!"

That was enough for us. We immediately put bars on all windows we were in the habit of opening. We didn't have to be personally held at knifepoint to get the message. And we hope that you personally don't have to develop diabetic retinopathy (eye damage) or neuropathy (nerve damage) or a diabetes-related cardiovascular problem or impotence to get the message that it's time to acknowledge that you've been in denial and that you should start accepting your diabetes and taking charge of it.

Now, let's explore some more of the many facets of denial, beginning with a basic denial: refusing to tell people that you have diabetes. In view of modern-day openness about health problems, why do certain people want to keep their diabetes hidden? They may not hide their diabetes from themselves, but they certainly try to keep it from everyone else. We've known married men who wouldn't even tell their wives about their diabetes. (How they managed that we'll never know!) How can these diabetic closet cases become secure and emotionally comfortable enough to reveal what they seem to consider their guilty secret?

Dr. Rubin: You're right that some people really hesitate to tell others about their diabetes. It took one man I know 49 years to tell anyone other than his wife and his doctors that he had diabetes. A woman didn't tell her teenage children for 7 years, and when she did, it was only because her blood sugars got so out of control that she needed to be hospitalized and couldn't hide it from them any longer.

Here are some of the reasons for not telling that I often hear.

1. Some people see diabetes as a weakness, especially when they're having trouble controlling it, and they don't like revealing their weaknesses. They may also be afraid of being a burden to others.

2. Some people have been taught to be secretive. This is especially true of those who developed diabetes as children 20 or 30 years ago when people tended to be more closed-mouth about almost everything. We talked less openly about sex, money, and diseases, including diabetes.

3. Occasionally diabetes is hidden for a religious reason. A woman I saw in a clinic grew up in a Christian Science family in a small town in North Carolina. Since church doctrine held that diabetes should be treated by prayer alone, her parents resolved to keep her insulin therapy a strict family secret. They took her to a doctor miles from where they lived. One day she had a serious insulin reaction at school and she got so scared that she

confessed to the school nurse that she took insulin. The nurse called her mother, and when she got home the little girl was spanked and yelled at for telling the nurse.

4. Some people keep quiet about diabetes because they have had bad experiences with revelation. This usually takes the form of some kind of work-related discrimination or intrusion by busybody "kind souls."

No matter what the reason for secrecy, being completely closeted is probably bad for you physically and psychologically. It's dangerous to have no one know you're diabetic, especially if you take insulin and are subject to hypoglycemic reactions. Most people who lock up their diabetes inside also feel emotionally uncomfortable. They tell me they often feel ashamed and isolated.

While complete closeting is almost always the wrong approach, there's no single right approach. Those of you who take insulin need to answer this question: Who needs to know about your diabetes in order to minimize the risk of acute problems like hypoglycemic reactions? As a general rule, family members, good friends, and at least one person you feel close to at work should be informed about your diabetes. These people need to know the signs of an insulin reaction and how to help you deal with one. Since there will be times when none of these people is around, you also need to carry some form of identification as a diabetic, so you'll get the right help quickly if you need it.

Beyond the requirements of safety, how open you should be about your diabetes is a purely personal matter. Some people like to be very open. They say it feels good to educate others, and they want people to know that if they are acting weird, it's probably because of diabetes rather than alcohol, drugs, or a serious attitude problem. Others want to talk about their diabetes (or even acknowledge its existence) only with very close friends. I can't say that one approach is right and the other wrong, because that's not the case. The only situations that concern me are those in which no one is told (because of the physical risk involved for the diabetic) and those in which people won't tell because they feel ashamed to be open.

If you want to be more open, the key is to become more comfortable with your diabetes. If you feel a little more comfortable, you'll probably be a little more open, and that will then probably help you feel a little more comfortable. These two things tend to reinforce each other positively.

June and Barbara: We could use a few hints here on how to go about breaking the ice. How do we start talking about diabetes and what do we say as an opening gambit?

Dr. Rubin: First, think about what you want to share and with whom. Is it fact or feelings you want to communicate? Is the person a co-worker, friend, or family member? In any case, you want conditions to be positive, so pick a time when you're relaxed and at ease, when you and the other person are feeling good about each other. Then just open the subject. Make it clear that you will be happy to talk more right now after you've said the main things you want to say, or are willing to continue the discussion later.

June and Barbara: If you've kept your diabetes a secret for a long period and suddenly decide to reveal it, that can have some surprising—even humorous—repercussions, as we read in *Diabetes: Caring for Your Emotions As Well As Your Health* by Jerry Edelwich and Archie Brodsky. They told the story of a woman named Denise who was diagnosed diabetic at the age of six; she had kept her diabetes a secret from virtually everyone.

> As she entered adult life, Denise found that deception generated more deception. After years of concealment, how could she suddenly say to someone, "I haven't told you all these years because I have this black hole in my otherwise well-adjusted life"? Her husband would prod

her, saying, "How about if we tell the so-and-sos the next time we see them?" But it was Denise's decision to make, and she held back.

What turned things around for Denise was having a baby. As she puts it, "I wasn't about to have a secret diabetic pregnancy.". . . When she [finally] told a long-time friend and co-worker first that she was pregnant and then that she had diabetes (all in the space of two minutes), he replied, "What else do you have to tell me? Are you gay too?"

Dr. Rubin: My son provided me with a wonderful example of how to be constructively revealing about your diabetes. He got an insulin pump during the summer just before his twelfth birthday. It was a large apparatus, not like the pocket-sized models they have now. He had to wear it on his belt out in plain view. Just before school started in September, I asked him what he was going to tell people when they asked about the contraption on his belt. He told me he had no idea what he would say.

After the first few days of class I asked him what he had done about explaining his pump. He replied, "I demonstrated the whole thing to Pip [his best friend]. I showed him the hold button, so he could turn off the insulin if I was having a reaction. I told Jason and Josh [two other good friends] that it was a medical device for my diabetes. When anyone else asked, I told them it was a Walkman."

Perfect! He insured his safety, and decided just how much he wanted each person in his life to know.

June and Barbara: A couple of forms of denial seem to be more common among men, as we'll discuss in the "Help for Those Who Want to Help Diabetics" section at the end of this chapter. But one form seems to be more common among women: not taking care of your diabetes because everyone else in the family must be cared for first. This is the old "I always come last" syndrome. What's going on here, and how can women suffering from this syndrome get their priorities straight?

Dr. Rubin: The "I always come last" syndrome is frighteningly common among diabetic women, especially older ones. One woman told me she was constantly preoccupied with the medical problems of her husband and her parents, but neglected herself something awful. Another said she was raised to take care of other people first and herself only if she had anything left over. A third woman denied her diabetes because her husband got upset whenever something was wrong with her.

Conditioning and a high degree of sensitivity to the feelings of others contribute to this syndrome. A woman who always puts herself last believes that her family expects, needs, demands, or can't survive without her complete dedication to their well-being. She may also have a lot of confidence in her ability to care for her family and very little in her ability to care for her diabetes. This only reinforces the syndrome.

Putting yourself last really means putting *everyone* last, contrary to what it may seem. Though you think you're sacrificing yourself for others, you're really rendering yourself incapable of doing anything for anyone. One woman described her attachment to this approach as playing Russian roulette with her diabetes. She's right. Even if the only thing that matters to you is the well-being of your loved ones, you must admit that your ability to help them ends if you're incapacitated or dead.

It's essential that you start giving yourself some of the loving attention you have always lavished on others. Your family will probably be more enthusiastic about this than you might imagine. After all, they love and need you. In fact, you'll probably find more resistance within yourself than you'll get from them. If so, keep reminding yourself that the best way to care for your loved ones is to stay healthy and live a long life.

June and Barbara: Occasionally we hear of someone who denies diabetes because he or she claims that no one in the family takes it seriously. They all seem to pretend that diabetes isn't there. Can you offer any help to diabetics in this predicament?

Dr. Rubin: This isn't a common situation, though I do hear of it from time to time. There's almost always a kernel of truth in the claim these diabetics make that their loved ones deny their diabetes. They say that no one makes allowance for it in family activities, that people act as if the diabetic should be able to do everything without accommodation for the disease, that feeling tired or sick generates an angry reaction from the family.

I know these family reactions are real and hard to deal with. At the same time, I think that when diabetics claim they can't deal with diabetes because of reactions like these, they're not facing the truth: that the critical factor in no one wanting to deal with their diabetes is their *own* denial, not their family's. Once they work through this using some of the techniques we've talked about in this chapter, they will find a way to deal with their family's unconstructive attitudes. Often a family's denial simply melts away, especially if they've been taking their cue from the diabetic all along. Even if they continue to put up roadblocks, the diabetic will be clear that his or her responsibility to himself or herself does not depend upon the family's acknowledgment of it.

June and Barbara: Do people with diabetic family members who have had severe complications or even died from the disease experience more denial that those who have no family history of diabetes? Dr. Lois Jovanovic-Peterson believes that her acceptance perhaps took too long because she had witnessed her father die blind and bedridden at the age of 50 after 20 years of diabetes. In her introduction to *The Diabetic Woman,* she wrote, "I saw my father crippled by the disease, and thus it was terrifying to me."

Another woman revealed this: "My sister died of diabetes at 33 years old. She died in my arms, and I was diagnosed exactly one year later. I've never gotten over her death, and I've never accepted my own diabetes, though I've had it for 12 years now."

Dr. Rubin: I have no hard evidence that denial is more common in these cases, but the fact that it exists at all is striking. You'd think that a traumatic experience with diabetic complications in a family member would scare anyone into doing everything to avoid the same fate. Unfortunately, it doesn't work that way. Maybe this kind of trauma makes some diabetics feel hopeless, not motivated. They've seen a loved one fall, and they can't shake the belief that the same will happen to them. We should remember that it was almost impossible to maintain good control and avoid complications 20 or 30 years ago, when the basic beliefs of many present-day diabetics were being established. People with no experience of those "bad old days" may actually be more optimistic and, therefore, more motivated to face up to their disease.

What can you do if you were traumatized by your experiences with diabetic family members? First, acknowledge to yourself how painful and frightening these experiences were—and still are. Next, look at how these experiences colored your beliefs about diabetes. If you're in denial, your beliefs are probably pessimistic, even absolutely fatalistic. For instance, you may believe that complications and early death are inevitable. Now you need to test the reality of these beliefs. They are not true in and of themselves. They are only true if you act in ways that create another self-fulfilling prophecy of the sort we discussed earlier.

You can create an opposite self-fulfilling prophecy if you put your mind to it. Today we know that good self-care leads to good blood-sugar control and that people who maintain good diabetes control are unlikely to suffer from diabetic complications.

June and Barbara: We'd like to really emphasize that, Dr. Rubin, because we've met so many people who cling to the dismal diabetes mythologies of the past and maintain a totally outmoded mind-set about their own choice in the future of their health. We think the scientific facts were pretty much summed up by a 1990 study reported in the *New England Journal of Medicine*. This was about diabetic retinopathy, the disease of the area in the back of the eye responsible for vision loss in diabetics. In this study glycohemoglobin tests (a blood test that measures overall blood-sugar control) were used to determine the degree of control. Severe retinopathy developed in only 2.9 percent of patients with glycohemoglobin levels below 8.4 percent (normal range), but in 44 percent of those with levels over 9.9 percent (higher than normal range). Those figures speak loud and clear. Why be one of the 44 percent who lose their vision when, by keeping your glycohemoglobin below 8.4 percent, the odds are that you can avoid diabetic vision loss?

Dr. Rubin: Agreed. We also have at our disposal an array of technological advances for improving diabetes control, and the number and effectiveness of these tools grow daily. In the 12 years since my son developed diabetes, the state of the art has gone from urine testing, fasting plasma glucose testing, and one shot of NPH insulin (long-range-acting insulin) to home blood-glucose monitoring, glycohemoglobin and fructosamine testing (both check overall control), and insulin pumps. On the horizon are blood-glucose testing that requires no finger sticks, and several forms of mechanical artificial pancreases. Now more than ever there's great wisdom in the words of Oliver Wendell Holmes, "The key to longevity is to develop a chronic, incurable disease and take good care of it."

The experience of diabetics who lived in the past need not be yours. Indeed, you have the power to ensure that it will not be.

June and Barbara: Have you had many patients who blame significant people in their lives for problems they have with their blood sugars or other aspects of their regime? In our growing collection of unorthodox diabetes syndromes, we might call this one the pass-the-buck syndrome. For instance, we've heard husbands say, "I can't follow my diet because my wife cooks too much food and I can't resist eating it if it's there." Or a woman might say, "I can't follow my diet because the family doesn't like the things I'm supposed to eat and I don't have the time and energy to cook two different meals." Even Dr. Lodewick, with whom we collaborated on *The Diabetic Man,* complained that his wife insisted on keeping Haagen-Dazs butter pecan ice cream in the house even though she knew it was irresistible to him.

Bosses are blamed for creating stressful situations that cause blood sugars to rocket. Health professionals are blamed for not spending enough time explaining how to handle diabetes. Children protest that if their parents would only get off their backs, they could handle their diabetes just fine.

In many cases the diabetic may be right. People around the diabetic do all sorts of detrimental things. But ultimately doesn't the buck of responsibility have to stop with the diabetic? If so, how does the diabetic avoid trying to pass it to someone else?

Dr. Rubin: Diabetes is a demanding disease. There are no breaks or holidays and it involves every aspect of your life, so it's no wonder that from time to time frustration boils over when things aren't going right. At those times you may feel an overwhelming desire to pass the buck.

There's always at least a bit of wisdom in your choice of buck-passing targets. Important people in your life can make it harder (or easier) for you to take good care of your diabetes. The boss who stays on your case *is* making it harder for you to avoid stress-induced blood-sugar elevations. The doctor you can't reach to discuss an insulin dose adjustment *is* making it harder for you to maintain good control. The loved one who insists on buying the only ice cream in the world that you absolutely cannot resist *is* making it harder for you to stay on a healthy diet.

Other people can make it harder for you to do the right thing, and if you want to blame them for that, you'll get no argument from me. But other people can't make it *impossible* for you to do the right thing. Only you can do that. So in all fairness, blaming other people for their transgressions should go hand-in-hand with accepting responsibility for the ultimate outcome. In fact, the issue goes beyond fairness to hard reality. If you depend on someone else to protect your health, you're not taking very good care of yourself and you are ultimately the one who will suffer.

So it's neither fair nor smart to pass the buck for your diabetes care. How can you avoid giving in to the temptation to do just that? First, you might find some relief in feeling justifiably angry about the fact that people are making your life harder (not impossible, remember, just harder). Blow off a little steam. Stomp and scream, if it helps you feel better. Once you've settled down a little, talk to the person about how you feel if you think there's any chance of a constructive outcome. That person is more likely to be open if you make it clear that he or she is not making your self-care impossible, only more difficult.

The one thing you don't want to do is sink back into buck-passing. There's simply too much at stake. Your relationship with the other person will suffer and so will your health. Worst of all, you'll never learn one of life's most wonderful lessons: that you have the power to overcome any obstacle that stands between you and good care of your diabetes.

June and Barbara: We've got another syndrome for you, one that's similar to passing the buck. We call this one the putting-iron syndrome because we originally noted it among golfers. In golf, putting is the most crucial and frustrating part of the game. If you're unable to putt well, you wind up with a high score. In golf as with blood sugar, high scores mean defeat and discouragement. Consequently, when a golfer's putting is off, he or she is likely to blame the putting iron for not getting the ball into the hole. Some golfers have been known to hurl away iron after iron in a fury, because "that [expletive deleted] putter ruined my game!"

We've seen the identical syndrome with equipment and products people use to play the even more challenging game of diabetes. When they get a high blood-sugar score, then "this meter isn't working right," or "this pump is fouling me up," or—June's favorite—"something's wrong with this insulin." When we used to teach the use of meters at the SugarFree Center, and we would prove beyond a reasonable doubt that a meter was functioning perfectly, some would still angrily throw the meter down, wanting to have nothing more to do with it, just like the golfers who throw away a good putter when they think it's what's making them go over par. What are your suggestions for treating this syndrome?

Dr. Rubin: You're right that it's related to the pass-the-buck syndrome. In both cases there may be some wisdom in passing the blame. Meters are not perfectly accurate or perfectly reliable. Insulin pump infusion sets do leak at times. Insulin does spoil occasionally and it sometimes acts in unpredictable ways. All of these things do happen, and when they do, your control suffers.

Then again, at other times you may think your meter or pump or insulin is to blame for your wacky blood sugars when it is not. That doesn't necessarily mean *you're* to blame, though. As much as we would all like to believe otherwise, diabetes management is not an exact science (or even exactly a science). Sometimes you can do everything by the book and get a result that makes no sense at all. Life with diabetes is like that. Not most of the time, fortunately, but some of the time, which feels like too much of the time.

June and Barbara: We'll say amen to that. So what to do?

Dr. Rubin: As with the pass-the-buck syndrome, I think it's fine to blow off a little steam. It's even safer here, because your meter or insulin is unlikely to get hurt feelings and yell back at you. Then you can play scientist. Try out your hypothesis that the equipment is to blame for your problem, that your blood sugar is not nearly as high as your meter says. Test your blood again, recalibrate your meter, use a different meter if you have another. Try a new bottle of insulin. Change over your insulin pump reservoir and infusion set. My son and I have often done this last, when we couldn't figure out a series of high blood sugars, even when there seemed to be nothing wrong with the equipment. Our motto was, "If things aren't going right, change over." Sometimes things straightened out. Was the changeover responsible? Who knows? I do know that it at least gave us the feeling we had some control over the situation, and that was good.

While you're playing scientist, you might want to turn your microscope on yourself. Think back over the events leading up to the problem that's bothering you. Did anything unusual happen? Did you eat, exercise, or medicate yourself any differently than usual? Did you undergo some unusual stress, physical or emotional? This kind of thinking might lead somewhere. Keep in mind, you're looking for a reason, not for something to blame.

If none of this investigatory brilliance bears fruit, the answer to your dilemma is probably that there is no answer to your dilemma. It's just one of those predictably unpredictable times that are best dealt with by simply letting them go or filing them away, as you prefer.

June and Barbara: Over the years we've had many diabetics ask us about certain "cures" for diabetes and even some who insisted they were controlling their blood sugars by eating nopal cactus, using herbal concoctions, or taking megadoses of chromium or zinc. When we first opened the SugarFree Center on a main street (originally it was in our home), there was an herbal product outlet across from our building. Not long after we put up our sign, the manager of the herb store came over to see what we did there. When we told him we were involved in diabetes care, with all confidence he announced, "Well, just send those diabetics over to me. We can cure them with our products." He handed June a brochure that gave a testimonial from a woman who had herbally lost 30 pounds and was "cured" of diabetes. We weren't surprised about six months later when he went out of business.

When people have come to us with their "cures" we've always had to let them down gently and even refuse to pass on their suggested treatments in our books. Sometimes no matter what we say, we can't dissuade them from their great faith in the remedy they're using. Are these beliefs in a cure a form of denial?

Dr. Rubin: Yes, believing that diabetes can be controlled or cured in unorthodox ways is a form of denial. So far as I know, none of these substances has a direct effect on diabetes, and using any of them as a substitute for a good diabetes regime is a risky business. But this form of denial isn't necessarily a bad thing, because using these substances can have an indirect benefit. If you believe in them, your denial can be the positive kind, possibly making you more relaxed and less stressed, and that can directly improve your blood-sugar control. In addition, you may feel more confident about your diabetes in general, and that could lead to better self-care and better control.

I try to approach so-called discoveries with an open mind. First, I'm always interested and excited. Then I ask myself about the potential costs and benefits of trying the new approach. Some new treatments are pretty benign and can simply be added to existing treatments. Others may have serious side-effects or are intended to replace existing treatments that have proved themselves. If the benefit/risk ratio seems good, I think about ways to reduce the risks even further. Finally, I want to know how people can tell if the new treatment is working and how a person will know when to stop the treatment. This is the approach I take because I want to be sure that our search for cures flows from positive denial and not from the negative kind.

June and Barbara: Here's an even more far-out one for you. Several years ago, we visited Sedona, Arizona, a center of popular belief in gems and their mystical powers. According to the people who believe in such things, different gemstones affect different parts of the body. The stone that's supposed to do great things for the pancreas and, hence, help diabetics is citrine quartz. Ever-ready to try something new, we got a couple of large citrine quartz pieces and put one on June's desk and one on the counter at the SugarFree Center to give off beneficial vibes.

One day an older gentleman came in and asked Melanie, an employee who's an aspiring actress with a great personality and wry sense of humor, what "that rock" was there for. Melanie answered straight-faced, "That cures diabetes."

The gentleman thought about this for a minute, then lowered his voice conspiratorially and asked, "How much do you want for it?"

Actually we thought for a while of offering small citrine quartz stones on a chain and calling them "placebo stones" to serve both to remind people to take good care of their diabetes and to give them the kind of positive outlook that you get when you read a good astrological forecast in the newspaper. We never did it, fearing that people would think of us as even kookier than we are—the Shirley MacLaines of diabetes—but we still don't think it's a bad idea. An article in the *New York Times* on the superstitions of business executives mentioned that "When executives wear their lucky clothes, they may somehow be empowered beyond their normal capabilities."

Of course, it's long been known that placebos can do a person a lot of good—showing even more the power of the mind in the mind/body connection. What do you think? Could a placebo help give a diabetic a better outlook on his or her life and disease and thereby promote acceptance?

Dr. Rubin: Absolutely. The key here is the feeling of confidence that certain objects, people, or situations provide. The way I think of it, this confident mood helps us reach our potential. When it comes to diabetes, I've seen placebo effects work in many wondrous ways.

Take a really mundane one for instance. Practically everybody believes they have a certain spot where shots hardly hurt at all, or a certain finger where sticking is much less painful, or a certain lancing device they claim is the only one to use. Different people swear by different spots or fingers or lancers, and that's the point (no pun intended). What works for you might not work for me, and a big part of the difference is mental. Does that make the effect any less real? I don't think so. Certainly not if we measure the effectiveness of a placebo by its power to help us do the right thing. A placebo generates confidence, confidence generates good self-care, good self-care generates good health, and good health generates more confidence. So a placebo can definitely be the catalyst for a positive cycle.

Placebos can help in another way, as well. If you feel more confident and relaxed, your whole physical system is in a more balanced state. You feel less stressed, and you're less likely to experience the direct negative effects of high stress levels on your diabetes. Many people say that their blood sugars shoot up when they're under stress. One patient of mine, Gary, uses an insulin pump. He says that on days his boss is out of town he can keep his blood sugars under good control on a basal rate of .52 units of insulin per hour. When his boss is in the office, he feels so stressed he has to raise his basal rate to .78 units per hour, and he still can't keep his blood sugars under 200 mg/dl! We've been working to help Gary control his stress, with only partial success. Maybe I should consider giving him a piece of citrine quartz—or, better still, a magic device he could use to make his boss disappear.

Placebos are popular in many fields that demand high performance. Major league baseball players have their lucky gloves and bats, for instance. It might seem paradoxical, but placebos probably work best when you recognize that the real power is coming from your mind, not from the glove or stone or lancing device.

Remember the story of Dumbo, the little elephant? He believed he could fly only if he clutched a crow's feather in his trunk. One day he was in a burning building—part of the circus act in which he performed—and he dropped his feather. He stood frozen with fear, the flames threatening to engulf him, until his friend Timothy Mouse convinced Dumbo that the power of flight lay within him (in his mind and enormous ears) and not in the feather he had lost. The feather let Dumbo experience his potential; it did not create that potential.

➤ Help for Those Who Want to Help Diabetics

June and Barbara: We've noticed an incredible amount of marital discord and tension when the diabetic spouse is in denial and the other spouse is frantic over the situation. It's most often wives who experience this kind of frustration when their husbands refuse to take care of their diabetes, ignoring it as if it didn't exist. These women go back and forth between screaming at their husbands and giving up completely. They complain that nothing they do makes any difference. Is there anything they *can* do?

Dr. Rubin: It's really hard to watch someone you love ignore his diabetes. Sometimes it looks so willful. It's like a take-off on the old Lesley Gore Song, "It's my body and I'll die if I want to!" But your loved one isn't really being willful. He's desperately struggling to avoid feeling overwhelmed. No one would bury his head in the sand for any other reason.

What can you do? First, recognize the painful (and sometimes stress-relieving) fact that you can't make your spouse face up to his diabetes. You don't have that much power or responsibility. Pushing him only creates a lot of tension and diverts you both from the real issue: *he* needs to find a way to stop acting like an ostrich.

One thing *you* can do is express your feelings. Tell him you are scared because his blood sugars are out of control and you are worried about the future. Tell him you love him and want to spend many happy, healthy years with him. Tell him you feel frustrated, helpless, and guilty about not being able to help him deal better with his diabetes. Please note that all of these are statements about how you feel. They are not judgments of his behavior. Your feelings are your responsibility; his behavior is his.

The other thing you can do is ask him to read the answers to the previous questions in this chapter. If you found this information interesting, say so, but don't push. If he picks up on it, you might talk together about his thoughts and beliefs and how to start doing things differently. Just remember how delicate this process is, and that your spouse has the only vote that counts when it come to deciding how far and how fast to move.

June and Barbara: We've had letters from wives and girlfriends of diabetic men who are distressed because the diabetic man won't let them have anything to do with his diabetes. He won't share his problems and won't talk about what's going on with his care. He almost seems to want to hide his diabetes from the one who is closest to him. What's the safest approach for a woman facing this situation?

Dr. Rubin: Diabetic men seem to shut out the women in their lives more often than diabetic women shut out their men. Maybe that's because men have been trained in stoicism more than women have. Men are more likely to see diabetes as a weakness or a burden to be borne in silence. Some men also stay closeted about their diabetes out of fear that loved ones may overprotect or police them.

Naturally, you can't make your mate open up about his diabetes. Pushing is self-defeating, because he has veto power over how much he shares with you. If he feels pressured, he'll probably clam up tighter. He'll only open up if he feels you're supporting him rather than pushing. Let's briefly review the guidelines for offering support, as they apply to fostering communication.

1. **Ask questions.** The key day-to-day question here is, "How's the diabetes going lately?" Ask this in a tone of

open, loving curiosity (this tone can be hard to maintain at times, I know). Sooner or later it's likely to get the ball rolling.

Another question might be, "Do you ever feel like talking about your diabetes and not do it?" If he says he sometimes does, the follow-up question might be, "Why do you think that happens?" You might also ask, "Is there anything I'm doing that gets in the way of our talking about diabetes?"

2. **Talk about your feelings.** Tell him how much you love him, how you worry about him, how you appreciate it when he talks openly about his diabetes. Be clear in your own mind and in what you say to him that you are expressing your feelings, not trying to influence his behavior. This might sound like a subtle distinction or even an untruth, but this kind of clarity is the only sound basis for communication. If your partner feels that he has responsibility for your feelings, he'll retreat deeper into silence. If, on the other hand, he feels you're simply being open with him, you'll be doing everything you can to encourage him to do the same.

3. **Accept the slowness of the communication process.** It takes time to build trust; actually, much more time than it takes to destroy it. You're both learning new ways to talk to each other. You can't develop a climate of openness overnight. Accept the small steps as successes and the big steps will follow. With patience, persistence, and practice, you can create the communication you need to support your life with diabetes.

June and Barbara: Not sharing your diabetes with family members is one form of denial, but the opposite approach—expecting some family member to take over all the responsibility for handling your diabetes—is another. How can this particular form of denial be overcome? It seems to be somewhat like the co-dependency situation we read so much about these days.

Dr. Rubin: Here, again, sex roles tend to make this a more common problem when the diabetic is a man. In our society caretaking is a skill more highly developed in women than in men.

Sometimes the diabetic is very open about wanting to have someone else manage his disease. One man told me he had turned his diabetes over to his wife because, "She does enough worrying for both of us." Another said he took it for granted his wife would carry his supplies when they went out, because "she has a big bag that she takes everywhere anyway." I'm the first one to approve when I see people providing their diabetic loved ones with lots of support. At the same time, it's important to make a distinction between supporting and what I call pallbearing, or carrying someone as if he were dead.

All too often, when a diabetic turns over responsibility for his care to his mate, she tends to feel like a pallbearer. A woman told me that she felt scared and angry at the burden she was bearing. Another echoed this sentiment, adding, "I feel completely responsible, which leads to a lot of panic and resentment." Taking complete care of someone else's diabetes simply does not work, no matter how hard you try. First of all, you're not with the person 24 hours a day, and even if you were you wouldn't be inside his body. You can't know what's going on in there. Second, it's exhausting to try to be someone else's pancreas. Finally, if you try to pallbear your husband, your relationship will suffer. Both of you will feel resentful and alienated. Eventually your relationship will devolve from wife-husband to parent-child or policeperson-criminal.

The solution to this dilemma is to start talking about it. Statements such as "I'm feeling like a policeperson" are generally better than ones like "You're taking no responsibility at all for your diabetes." Discuss what it means to be supportive, what it means to be a pallbearer, and what it means to be a policeperson. Look at the pros and cons of each approach. Acknowledge your loved one's interest in having you share responsibility and even his interest in escaping responsibility altogether. These are perfectly normal feelings; they're only a problem if they form the foundation for how he deals with his diabetes.

In general, it's best for the two of you to express interests rather than taking positions, because this leads to cooperation rather than confrontation. For instance, taking a position is saying, "I refuse to keep reminding you to test your blood." The resulting battle may be out in the open or under the surface, but, in either case, it will be painful and unproductive. You don't want this. A close, loving relationship means so much, especially when you are living with diabetes.

On the other hand, when you look at your interests together, you'll find that the most important ones are shared. You both have an interest in your spouse's health and in maintaining a good relationship. Your loved one is interested also in help and support. He doesn't want to feel alone and overwhelmed. You're also interested in not feeling overly responsible. If you can put all these interests on the table, along with any others you have, you'll probably find yourselves asking the right question: "How can we both get our needs met?" Now you're on the way to an agreement you can live with.

Remember that the agreements you make about how to live with diabetes are living agreements. It takes time for them to develop, and you'll need to adjust them as your interests change.

➤

OBSESSION
TOO MUCH OF A GOOD THING

Being preoccupied with your diabetes or going even further to become obsessed by it is the other side of the coin of denial. You might call it the heads side because your head is always full of thoughts of diabetes and your routines.

Of course it's a good thing to be serious and conscientious about keeping your diabetes in control, and it's a good thing to want to learn as much as you can about diabetes and to put all that you learn into practice. The philosopher Mae West once maintained that "Too much of a good thing can be wonderful," but when it comes to focusing on diabetes, too much of a focus may not be all that wonderful. It may not be wonderful to friends, relatives, and even casual acquaintances who aren't as enthralled with the condition as you are. They may become bored, irritated, and even exasperated by your monomaniacal preoccupation with your disease, by your refusal to make even minor variations in your diabetic routines, by your always putting yourself and your health needs first.

We once knew a man who was in business with a diabetic. When the business went through a bad period, the diabetic partner kept complaining that the stress of the business problems was sending his diabetes out of control. Every day he'd take multiple blood sugars and harangue his partner with the damage being done to his diabetes. The partner, who wasn't feeling any too good about the business himself, was often heard muttering, "How about *me?* Nobody seems to care about my blood pressure or the fact that I might be getting an ulcer. It's nothing but what this business is doing to his diabetes! I wish he'd shut up. I'm sick of it."

We must admit we feel that if you have to go one way or the other, being a tad obsessed is being better than being in denial—especially in the early days of your diabetes. We've known a number of people (present company included) who were—to say the least—preoccupied with their diabetes when they were trying to learn how to handle it. It all seems so confusing at first that you have to do a lot of reading, asking questions, and talking about it. We remember when June went on a ski trip just three days after going on insulin. She sat in the hotel dining room with a copy of *Food Portions Commonly Used* open on her lap, carefully analyzing each forkful she put in her mouth. But in a few months when she knew more about the diabetic diet, she was again a normal, nonpreoccupied dining companion.

In those early stages what appears to be talking to others may actually be a kind of talking to yourself, musing, as you try to sort out what to do from the as-yet-undigested collection of information that's been dumped on you.

Learning diabetes is something like learning to write poetry. In the beginning of verse-writing you have to study and practice using over and over the traditional verse forms—sonnet, Alexandrine, rondeau, ballade—until you have them down pat. They're the foundation of your art. Later on, when you've mastered these forms, you can abandon the rigid patterns and let yourself go with nontraditional and free verse. In diabetes you have to study and practice using over and over the standard therapies until you have them down pat. They're the foundation of your diabetes care. Later on when you've mastered these, you can let yourself go with nontraditional therapies that work well for you and make for a much freer life. But in the beginning it shouldn't be too surprising to anyone—including yourself—if you seem to be preoccupied with learning the art of diabetes.

So, as far as we're concerned, just as is true in most aspects of life, there's an upside as well as a downside to having a preoccupation or obsession with diabetes. We'll ask Dr. Rubin to help us explore both sides now.

—June and Barbara

June and Barbara: Maybe we should start with a little of the downside. Since we put in some good words for being a little preoccupied or obsessed with diabetes, what are the problems with that?

Dr. Rubin: It's easy to see why you might become preoccupied or obsessed with regimen precision, especially in the early stages. It gives you the comforting feeling that diabetes and its consequences can be perfectly controlled. It's a way of dealing with the deep down fear that every person with diabetes and every person who loves someone with diabetes experiences.

The unfortunate truth is that diabetes management is *not* an exact science, much as we would like to believe otherwise. Therefore, if you start out preoccupied-going-on-obsessed with your diabetes and you resolutely follow a rigid pattern of control, you're setting yourself up for tremendous disappointments down the line when blood sugar results don't reward your efforts by perfectly matching your expectations. You can get to the point where you crack instead of bending, and you just say, "To hell with it, no matter how hard I try nothing works," and give up trying to control your blood sugar.

A second problem with preoccupation or obsession is that it can make your existence an arid experience in which diabetes defines your life rather then being incorporated into it. You become what others may describe as a professional diabetic.

June and Barbara: When it comes to extremism in diabetes control, we can give an example which illustrates how it can go beyond defining your life and lead to even more dire consequences. Here is a letter we once received from the brother of a diabetic man who was a client of the SugarFree Center:

Dear Folks:
I received your mailing. I would like to bend your ear about what I hope is a very unusual occurrence.

My brother *was* a fanatic about controlling his sugar. Within a year he was testing 5 times a day and injecting 2 or 3 times a day. The only problem was that he cut it too close. In an effort to stave off future problems he ran very lean. The result was an increase in reactions and near reactions.

The night he died (at the age of 42) he ran his last test at 11:00 P.M. It showed 70. He never woke up. The autopsy was done by the county and showed nothing. His doctors said that his veins showed the least damage they had seen in a person with diabetes for 34 years. So, is it possible to be too careful? How do you spot a diabetic who will become obsessed about low blood readings?

Anyway, as better systems become available I hope those diabetics trying to do the best job of controlling sugar don't fall victim to their own good intentions.

Is there anything this man's brother could have done to help him avoid falling victim to his own good intentions?

Dr. Rubin: He would have had to persuade him to seek counseling to help him identify the basic fears that motivated such dangerous and fatal behavior. There are also medications which could have reduced the fear and preoccupation which ultimately drove him to his death.

Most people with milder forms of diabetes-related preoccupation can learn to deal with their problem on their own, using some of the suggestions we'll be discussing in this chapter.

June and Barbara: We've sometimes noticed a thoroughly nontoxic form of preoccupation with diabetes. In our syndrome-o-rama, we call it the engineer's syndrome because we've seen it most frequently in practitioners of that profession. They love working over the details of diabetes therapy, keeping meticulous records of their blood sugar and fine-tuning their control. It causes them no distress at all—it's like playing an intricate, infinitely satisfying game to them.

Our favorite manifestation of the engineer's syndrome occurred at an American Diabetes Association Annual Scientific Session in New York. We were talking with a well-known diabetic diabetologist who was, indeed, an engineer before he made a midlife career change to medicine. We were chatting with him between sessions when suddenly he said, "Excuse me, I have to go eat a handful of peanuts. I took a shot to cover them a while ago." He walked over, chomped down his peanuts, and casually returned to resume the conversation.

Later June was musing that if she had to be that meticulous in her diabetes control, it would drive her crazy—or maybe that should be nuts! Yet he seemed perfectly happy and relaxed with this kind of therapy, and no one can deny that he has superb control. This leads us to ask, how do you draw the line between being obsessed and good self-care?

Dr. Rubin: The line can't be drawn on the basis of how much time and thought you put into caring for your diabetes. Many people who put in lots of time and thought are clearly not obsessive and compulsive about it. (Obsessions are thoughts, and compulsions are actions triggered by those thoughts.) I distinguish good care from an obsessive-compulsive pattern on the basis of how comfortable or uncomfortable the process feels. If you are obsessed you feel tense, fearful, despairing, and driven almost all of the time. You are constantly preoccupied with all the horrible things that might happen to you and all the things you must do in a desperate attempt to avoid them. If you're simply taking good care of your diabetes, these feelings are rare or nonexistent. (Those happy, relaxed engineer's syndrome people would fall into this category.) You may often feel concerned, and as if you are stretching to live a normal life, but you almost never feel the extremes of distress that characterize obsession.

In addition to feeling uncomfortable, compulsive diabetes-related behavior tends to be rigid and inflexible. It focuses on form rather than results. In fact, it is often unrelated to any realistic goal. Even the person engaged in this kind of behavior usually recognizes that it is unreasonable and excessive. Because of all these characteristics, compulsive behavior often disrupts normal routines in other important areas of life—work, social life, and intimate relationships. A person who deals with diabetes compulsively might be attached to the habit of taking the same amount of insulin, always taking it at home (perhaps even in a certain place at home), at exactly the same time every morning and every evening. He can't vary this routine to take into account variations in blood sugar, so he is often over- or underdosing himself. And he can't take his insulin away from home, or a little earlier or later, so he deprives himself and his family and friends of many opportunities for shared good times.

Good care focuses on the goals of maintaining good diabetes control and a fairly normal life, and it is flexible in the pursuit of these goals. Good care makes the diabetes regimen a matter-of-fact (albeit crucially important) part of living, not a painful preoccupation that negates all other aspects of living.

June and Barbara: It looks as if we have here another tight-rope for diabetics to walk—the one between good care and a good life. All diabetics have times when what they think of as their diabetic "have to's" interfere with their life plans or needs. Of course, the converse can also be true. As we described in *The Diabetic Man,* when Dr. Lois Jovanovic was working with her family desperately fighting the fire that was about to engulf her Santa Barbara home, she didn't follow her customary meticulous diabetic routines. She realized she hadn't taken her pre-dinner injection and that the adrenaline of the crisis was probably driving her blood sugar into the stratosphere, so when there was a momentary break in the fire's intensity she ran inside and, without checking her blood sugar or even measuring her insulin, drew up a big dose, shot it in, and raced back to fight the fire.

The decision about what takes precedence usually isn't that clear-cut. It's not always easy to know when to put diabetes first and when to put your life needs and desires first—and you must make this decision constantly. What's the intelligent way to decide?

Dr. Rubin: Countless times each day diabetics are faced with a choice between "doing the right thing" and "living normally." Often the choice feels like a painful one between preoccupation and denial. How do you walk that tightrope between having diabetes rule your every move and living as if it had no importance at all? Here are a few guidelines:

1. Don't go to extremes. Any either/or approach to living with diabetes is doomed to failure. You can't maintain it over time because it's unbalanced. Balance is vital when you're walking a tightrope!
   Don't try to be perfect. You'll never get there, and you'll drive yourself—and everyone else—crazy if you try. Diabetes control isn't about perfection. It's about good control. On the other hand, don't try to deny your diabetes. It only gets worse if you do. It reminds me of an auto air filter commercial on TV. The mechanic says, "You can pay me now (a little) or you can pay me later (a lot!)."

2. Accept—on faith at first, if you have to—the fact that every situation presents a choice that respects both the needs of your diabetes and your need to live a fairly normal life. At first you will probably have trouble identifying these choices, or even believing that they exist. But with practice, you will get better and better at making them.

3. Devote yourself to identifying the kinds of balanced choices I've just mentioned. This does take work, and for most people it's as demanding as learning a new language or how to bat lefty if you're right-handed, but the rewards are beyond measure. The amount of energy required is actually a lot less than you use trying to maintain an either/or approach of obsession or denial.

4. The clearest way to tell whether you're making a balanced choice is by how you feel. If you're making a balanced choice, you feel pretty comfortable and at peace. You may feel some disappointment, which is natural, but you don't feel the intense discomfort and distress that accompany an unbalanced choice.

June and Barbara: We still face the major problem of how to make these balanced choices.

Dr. Rubin: The key is working with your Sympathetic Scientist. You have one dwelling inside you—we all do. This inner voice approaches difficult situations rationally and lovingly, gently searching for explanations and offering suggestions for the present and the future. All you have to do is listen.

In this situation, the Sympathetic Scientist will guide you by asking you a few simple questions:

➤ What's the choice you're making here?
➤ What are the benefits of this choice?
➤ What are the drawbacks of this choice?
➤ Based on your answers so far, are you satisfied with your choice or would you like to consider an alternative?
➤ If you'd like to consider an alternative, can you think of any with more benefits or fewer drawbacks?

The fun of working this way is that once you get the ball rolling, it really does roll.

June and Barbara: Boy, does it! We vividly remember one particularly dramatic diabetic ball-rolling June had back when she was a novice of only a couple of years of diabetes. She'd been on insulin only one year. Her dosage was the then-standard one shot of NPH a day.

We were in Courchevel, France, on a two-week ski trip. June was having two major problems. First, she had bouts of hypoglycemia almost daily, especially around 6:00 P.M., because of the blood-sugar-lowering effect of the skiing coupled with the stretched-out French dining hours. Her routine was to get up at 6:30 A.M., inject NPH insulin, breakfast at 7:30 A.M., and have dinner at 8:30 P.M. (The dining room doors didn't even swing open for dinner until 8:00 P.M.) You can see the flaw. NPH insulin peaks in eight to ten hours. This preprogrammed her to eat dinner at 5:00 or 6:00 as she did at home. During those late-afternoon low-blood-sugar bouts, she had to feed her insulin a bunch of sweets to keep herself sane and functioning.

That brings us to the second problem. Dinner was a beautiful and elaborate feast—appetizer, main course, cheese tray, fruit, and dessert. And it was a feast that was already paid for since we had booked half-pension at the hotel. But by the feast time, June had used up her insulin peak with snacks to control the blood sugar, so there was little of it left to handle dinner. If she did more than pick at her food, she'd get raging high blood sugars.

What to do? If she had gone to one extreme, she might have said, "Diabetes comes first" and eaten something more substantial than snacks at 6:00—perhaps a sandwich purchased when cafés were open at noon. Then she would have skipped dinner, leaving Barbara without a dining companion and herself without the pleasure of a lovely French meal. Or she could have gone to the other extreme and said, "I'm only here for two weeks and I'm going to enjoy myself and eat whatever I want for dinner. I don't care how high it raises my blood sugar."

Just as Dr. Rubin advises, she did neither. She consulted her Sympathetic Scientist—although she didn't even know she had one at the time. Her Sympathetic Scientist reminded her of the time she had the flu the previous year and couldn't stay in control. Her doctor had put her on booster shots of Regular insulin before lunch and dinner. That worked instantly and effectively to bring her blood sugar down.

As luck would have it, June had packed Regular insulin just to be on the safe side in case she got the flu, a cold, or some other infection on the trip. Her Sympathetic Scientist developed a theory of how she could have normal blood sugar (no lows and no highs) and eat her evening feast as well. All she had to do, the SS reasoned, was switch to Regular insulin, dividing her daily dosage of 12 units of NPH into 6 units of Regular before breakfast, 3 before lunch, and 3 before dinner. Although Regular's range of action is only about six hours, the SS figured that in spite of the long stretch with no insulin between 2:00 A.M. and 6:30 A.M., and the short period before dinnertime, she wouldn't have high blood sugar before breakfast or dinner, thanks to the marvelous stabilizing and carry-over effect of the intense exercise of all-day skiing. The SS was right!

The rest of the trip went beautifully—superb meals and no more worry about before-dinner hypoglycemia. On the flight home, she got a fringe benefit: she had fewer problems with the odd dining schedule and the time-zone changes. It was as if she'd suddenly been given back the freedom to live as she wanted to.

On her return from the trip, she went back on NPH for a short time, but she no longer had patience with its inflexibility, so she popped the question to her doctor: "Would it be okay with you if I changed to three shots of Regular insulin a day?"

His answer was unequivocal. "The more shots you take, the better control you have. I wish I could get all my diabetic patients to go on Regular, but only two or three are willing to inject themselves more than once a day. I don't even suggest it to them anymore."

Of course, since she didn't exercise as intensely at home during her workaday life, she and her doctor adjusted the dosage accordingly, even adding a little NPH so she wouldn't get up in the morning with high blood sugar. (Several years later she dropped NPH and started using ultralente, which doesn't peak but provides an all-day, all-night, ongoing basal dose.)

Thus, by avoiding extremes and an either/or approach, June (or, rather, her Sympathetic Scientist) was able both to live the kind of freewheeling life she loves and to do the right thing for her diabetes. In fact she was able to do the best thing possible for her diabetes. Since this was about six years before the multiple-injection theory came into vogue, she had that much additional time of tight control in her diabetic life. This may in great part account for the fact that she has absolutely no complications after 25 years of diabetes.

Dr. Rubin: Not all ideas you and your Sympathetic Scientist come up with will be an unqualified success like this one. Some of the new ideas will be terrible and some will be only okay. But keep in mind the fact that even a really good idea will be a compromise. That's the hallmark of balanced choices.

Two things make this process effective. First, it opens things up, generating lots of options for any given situation. Second, it clarifies the fact that you're making a *choice*. When you see that you're choosing and not being forced to do something, that awful, tense, fearful feeling will lift, to be replaced by a feeling of peace and self-control.

There are no right or wrong choices, only ones that work or don't work for you. Once you and your Sympathetic Scientist have done your thing, you can trust your decision, but that doesn't mean the decision is cast in concrete. In fact, the best choices are flexible ones. You try them out to see how they feel, evaluating and adjusting them as needed.

If you find you're having lots of trouble making balanced choices, and your Sympathetic Scientist seems to be out to lunch, consider getting some outside help. You might turn to a support group or to a counselor who understands diabetes.

June and Barbara: Now we come to something that we've particularly noticed: some diabetics seem to be obsessed not so much with sweating over meticulous diabetes control, but simply with talking about diabetes all the time. Their control may or may not be meticulous. We may be at fault here because we encourage people to tell us about their diabetic adventures and misadventures. We find them fascinating. We hang upon their tales as Scheherazade's sultan must have hung on hers. Many of these people may not talk about diabetes nearly as much with others as they do with us. It's just that it's probably so rare for diabetics to find someone who is genuinely interested in every little up-and-down-and-in-and-out detail of their disease that they take full advantage of the situation.

On the other hand, we have had intimates of diabetics sidle up to us and say something like, "All Ted seems to want to do is discuss his diabetes. He talks about it to anyone and everyone to the point that he's getting to be a bore on the subject. What can I do to get him to cut it out?"

Would talking about diabetes be an example of obsession and, if so, how do people go about getting their minds—and mouths—off the subject?

Dr. Rubin: I don't have as much experience with this problem as you do. When I have a diabetic patient, of course diabetes is what we talk about almost exclusively. In a clinical situation if the patient didn't want to talk about diabetes, *that* would be a problem.

I've actually known very few people who talk about their diabetes a lot outside of a small circle that includes family and friends—although they could overdo it in that small circle. I assume there's some hyperbole in the image of a diabetic talking about his condition to anyone and everyone, so here's the issue I'll address: a diabetic who talks a lot about the disease.

Talking about diabetes this way could be considered compulsive, not obsessive. Obsessions are thoughts, and compulsions are actions triggered by those thoughts. Whether the talk is compulsive depends less on the amount of time the diabetic talks or the number of people addressed than on the quality of the communication. Since communication involves both sending and receiving information, we need to look at the communication from the perspective of the diabetic and of the listener.

June and Barbara: What would be the earmarks of noncompulsive communication?

Dr. Rubin: Talking about your diabetes is probably not compulsive if you're feeling alive, comfortable, and in control as you are talking. (It's possible to feel this way even if the topic is something painful.) You can also steer clear of compulsive talking if you try to keep your audience in mind. Is what you're saying relevant to this person? You can gauge the relevance in a number of ways. Were you asked a question? Does this person have a personal connection to diabetes? Is there some reason you want to educate him or her? Talking about diabetes is also noncompulsive if the length and intimacy of the communication fits your relationship with the person you're addressing.

June and Barbara: How can you tell if you've slipped over the border into compulsive diabetes talk?

Dr. Rubin: Talking about your diabetes *can* be compulsive if:

1. You feel agitated and pressured as you talk.

2. You find yourself talking about your diabetes to people for whom this information seems to have no relevance.

3. You tend to tell the same story over and over again whenever you talk about your diabetes.

If you find that you're talking compulsively, do yourself a favor and don't burden the people around you. Look for signals that this is a compulsive communication: the person you're talking to will say very little, avoid eye contact, check the time, move a little farther away from you. If you see these signs, respond appropriately by wrapping up the conversation. Then find another way to deal with the obsessions that trigger this compulsive talking. Consult your Sympathetic Scientist, join a support group, find a counselor.

June and Barbara: Here's another syndrome for you to analyze. We call it the great pretender syndrome because those who have it pretend they're more preoccupied with diabetes than they really are. For example, June has sometimes found herself insisting that her diabetes does not allow her to participate in certain social or recreational activities that someone else wants her to participate in. Sometimes she even uses diabetes to get out of eating something that's perfectly acceptable on her diet but that she doesn't particularly care for.

When she considers what she's doing in the cold light of reason, she suspects that many times she's simply using her diabetes to get out of doing something she'd rather not do. Diabetes is a convenient excuse. No one can argue with you when you appear to be a conscientious (preoccupied? obsessed?) diabetic taking good care of your disease. Deep down June knows she could probably work around the problem if she really wanted to. Do other diabetics engage in this great pretension in their family, social, and work situations?

Dr. Rubin: Yes, I think this is pretty common. In fact, using chronic physical complaints to get out of things we'd rather not do is nearly universal. Think about the times you've used your bad back, your allergies, or even your spouse's bad back or allergies to avoid some commitment. I guess we all tend to feel an illness is the most convenient and acceptable excuse on these occasions.

This reminds me of my own growing up, where the rule was, "You can stay home if you have a fever." Properly motivated, I developed a simple but effective system for generating a fever: I vigorously rubbed the thermometer on my sheet. This would generally get me a reading of about 107°, and I would then shake the temperature down to some plausible level. My career in personal fever control came to a dramatic conclusion one day when my mother returned to my room before I had a chance to complete my task. When she saw the reading of 106.7°, she nearly fainted. Faced with a choice between confessing right away or later at the hospital to which my mother was preparing to rush me, I chose the former.

My efforts to use illness as an excuse were completely conscious, but most times it's not that way if you're diabetic.

Often you don't feel well, and this feeling of unwellness tends to grow almost unconsciously when there's something unpleasant on the agenda.

June and Barbara: Conscious or not, it sounds as if using illness as an excuse can sometimes serve as a safety valve when "the world is too much with you." After all, if you didn't have diabetes, you could always dig up some other reason to get out of something you didn't want to do.

Dr. Rubin: Yes, using diabetes as an excuse (or reason, as the case may be) has some things to recommend it. First of all, it's handy and effective; it generally gets you out of whatever it is you want to avoid without a major hassle. Most people understand. Second, maybe you really do need to give yourself a break; there might be some wisdom in the feeling that you want to skip the activity. You may have a tough time letting yourself off the hook on any basis other than your diabetes. Third, it's nice to know that your diabetes is good for *something*.

June and Barbara: On the other hand, handy though it may be, there must be something to dis-recommend this diabetic social extrication device.

Dr. Rubin: Of course, there are disadvantages to using diabetes this way. In the first place, you may be avoiding experiences that could be interesting, rewarding, fun, good for you, or positive in some other way. In the second place, if you don't acknowledge the real reasons why you're avoiding the situation, you may stay confused in your own mind about what is really going on, and you'll get no practice developing the valuable skill of just saying, "No, thank you."

If you convince yourself that it's the diabetes alone that's standing in your way, your sense of being burdened will increase, even when it comes to things you want to do. Finally, if you use this excuse a lot, people around you will begin to see your diabetes as a more serious problem than it is, and you as more seriously afflicted than you are.

June and Barbara: How do you decide how and when to say no, how and when to use your diabetes as the excuse or reason?

Dr. Rubin: All you have to do is consult your Sympathetic Scientist and answer these questions the SS puts to you:

1. Do you have any reason other than your diabetes for saying no? Maybe you're shy, don't like the activity, need a "mental health" day, or whatever.

2. How much of your wish to say no comes from this other reason? Is it 1 percent, 50 percent, 99 percent?

3. Is there some way to minimize your diabetes-related reasons for saying no?

4. Do you want to change your mind and say yes, now that you have answered questions two and three? Maybe you can now see how to take care of your diabetes and enjoy the activity. Maybe you want to overcome your shyness and Just Do It.

5. Do you want to acknowledge to the people involved your other reasons for saying no? This would be an opportunity to face these other issues directly or to suggest alternative activities that you might prefer.

The goal in all of this is to make sure your choice is a conscious one. Conscious choices are always the best. They take into account all the facts, and they're much easier to live with.

June and Barbara: To end our discussion of preoccupation and obsession on a high note, we want to mention a number of diabetics who have a magnificent obsession. They become so involved with diabetes and so knowledgeable about it that they decide to devote their careers to it. Our favorite example of this is Ron Brown, our first employee back when we started the SugarFree Center.

Ron had been diagnosed in his senior year at college and resolutely (obsessively?) read everything he could find on the subject, ranging from our books to the most abstruse medical tomes and journals. When he came home for summer vacation, while he waited for graduate school to begin—he planned to work for a graduate degree in psychology—he hied himself over to see us and convinced us that we needed some help and that he was the man for the job.

He had an instant rapport with the diabetic clients, and it didn't take him long to realize that he really loved helping people with their problems in dealing with the disease. Since the aspect with which they seemed to need the most help was diet and since he was a talented cook, he abandoned his psychology degree plans and enrolled in the dietitian program at the University of California at Berkeley. He then worked as a Registered Dietitian (R.D.) for a few years at Scripps Clinic in San Diego, giving dietary counseling to diabetes patients and later on even helping them with their insulin therapy. Since he was so knowledgeable about diabetes and since he wore a white coat, patients assumed he was a doctor and started calling him Dr. Brown. Before long, he decided to make it a legitimate title and began taking the necessary premed courses.

Because of Ron's unique background and experience, he was accepted by a number of major medical schools—including his first choice—despite the fact that he was an elderly gentleman of 30. You'll be happy to know that in his interviews, his diabetes seemed to be more of an asset than a hindrance in his quest for admission.

We just received an invitation to his graduation at the University of California, Davis. He'll soon start his residency and in three years he'll be in practice specializing in helping diabetics—and he'll be the only diabetic dietitian-physician in the country and probably in the world. He freely admits that if it hadn't been for his diabetes, he wouldn't be a doctor today.

Although Ron is deeply involved with diabetes, he's certainly not obsessed by it as he was when we first knew him. Then he could hardly think or talk about anything else. These days he's more likely to want to discuss travel, skiing, gourmet cooking, wine, or his wife or baby daughter.

Every time we go to a diabetes conference we're struck by how many diabetics have turned their magnificent obsession with diabetes into a career of helping others as nurses, dietitians, physicians, exercise therapists, social workers, or psychologists. We're also struck by the fact that they, like Ron, have their diabetes in perspective and their minds focused on the productive activities and joys of their lives.

➤ Help for Those Who Want to Help Diabetics

June and Barbara: In Bernie Siegel's book, *Peace, Love and Healing,* he says, "Sometimes the illness is so effective at getting the sick person the care and attention he needs that everyone around him is exhausted by the effort of meeting those needs. In physical diagnosis there is something I call 'Siegel's Sign,' when a family comes into my office with everybody looking sick except for one individual, I know that the one who looks well is the one with the illness. That one person is manipulating and controlling everyone else."

Dr. Rubin, have you noticed "Siegel's Sign" in many of your diabetics and their families? Have the families become the obsessed ones about the condition, and look the worse for wear because of it?

Dr. Rubin: I can't say that I've had much experience with "Siegel's Sign." In general, people who use their illness to manipulate and control their families are in pretty bad physical shape themselves. In fact, it's their desperate shape that motivates the family to sacrifice so much in the first place. The sacrifice seems to be born of a deep and abiding love; there's rarely any tension about it. This kind of attention is what we mental-health types call secondary gain. It's the silver lining that comes with the cloud of serious physical problems.

In most cases I see, this pattern develops when some serious diabetic complication arises and a previously vigorous person is laid low. Then I notice that the physical recovery is much more drawn-out and complicated than it is usually. The person may become a near-invalid and stay that way for months on end, lovingly tended to by children, spouse, and parents. When I talk to the diabetic, I almost always find that he or she was a very strong, independent, "good little soldier" type of person from childhood—exactly the opposite of now.

More talk generally reveals two things: first, the person didn't get as much nurturing as needed growing up; and second, that's exactly the need being met now. Being an invalid has the benefit of drawing upon the love and support that wasn't forthcoming years ago. I have no way to explain why the very parents who couldn't cherish their children when they were young can do it when they are ill adults, but I've seen it happen again and again. It's beautiful in a way, but it also tends to keep the diabetic an invalid, because recovery means giving up all these goodies. I guess the parents may also be recovering something they lost.

June and Barbara: How do you resolve this dilemma? You don't want to cut off the love that the diabetic needs most—and that perhaps you need most to give—yet you don't want to contribute to prolonging the invalid state.

Dr. Rubin: It takes several steps. First, you have to identify the problem of conflict around dependence, and its roots in childhood. Second, you have to acknowledge that the person's incapacity is based in part on the fact that illness draws the long-yearned-for loving care. Third, you have to be clear that while the need to be cared for is very strong and totally legitimate, the form it is taking has too many negative consequences. Finally, you need to identify and practice new ways to draw upon the wonderful love and caring concern the family is showing, ways that encourage health rather than incapacity. While this process usually takes time, it almost always concludes beautifully, with everyone involved stronger and closer than ever before.

June and Barbara: Let's hearken back to our discussion of the situation in which the diabetic person is constantly talking compulsively (and boringly!) about diabetes. How can intimates of a diabetic protect themselves and others from the seemingly endless preoccupation with diabetes?

Dr. Rubin: Naturally, the audience has a responsibility in this situation. If diabetics talk compulsively about their diabetes, people they don't know well will just avoid them. Those of you who are close to a diabetic don't have that choice. You need to take a direct approach.

To begin with, you should stay as open as you possibly can to what the diabetic has to say. That's what being there for another person is all about. At the same time, you can't really be there if you're feeling completely fed up. This is a particularly difficult situation because you're probably deathly afraid of hurting the diabetic's feelings. Still, you have to take some kind of stab at the subject. Maybe something along the lines of, "I feel so sad when you tell me again and again about how hard your diabetes is. And I guess I feel frustrated, too. I want to be able to do something or at least say something that helps, but I can't. It feels like we're both kind of stuck—you with your diabetes and me with my inability to help you."

This might start a different and more creative conversation, or it might go in one ear and out the other, never making contact with a single brain cell. Even if the latter happens, you've still accomplished something. You've spoken up, and most people who speak up tell me it's a relief.

If your compulsively talkative diabetic is a family member or very close friend, you may need to go beyond simply speaking up, if that doesn't work. You may need to say that you can't take it anymore; that you listen and listen and listen and you always hear the same thing, and you think that's bad. It's bad for you, bad for your loved one, and bad for your relationship. Suggest that you find another, more constructive and productive way to talk about diabetes, or suggest that you go to a support group together—and do it!

CHAPTER 3

ANGER
YOUR PERFECT RIGHT

According to David Burns, M.D., author of *Feeling Good,* one of the reasons for anger is a feeling that a situation is unfair. What could be more unfair than having diabetes? You did nothing to deserve it, yet here it is with you for your whole life, causing restrictions, creating risks, costing you buckets of money, making you stick yourself with a lancet and, in some cases, an insulin needle. It's rotten and absolutely unfair. You have every right to be angry.

Psychologist Willard Gaylen holds the theory that another cause of anger is a feeling that you don't have control of a situation. You don't have perfect control of your diabetes and you never will no matter how hard you try. You have every right to be angry.

You're a human being and therefore subject to all the normal life situations that everyone else is subject to—the neighbors who keep you awake at night, the child (or parent or spouse) who drives you up the wall, the arrogant, demanding boss or the lackadaisical, lazy, unreliable employee, traffic and the rude, even life-threatening drivers crashing around in it, politicians, taxes, the outrageous and often incorrect bills you receive, the stupidity and greed that are rife in our society. Your diabetes doesn't make you immune to any of these outrages. You have every right to be angry.

But having a right doesn't mean you're required to exercise it. If you're waiting to cross the street and the light turns green, you have every right to step off the curb and march to the other side, but if you see a car barreling toward you against the light at 80 miles an hour, you'd be a fool to step into its path. You'd be a fool to exercise your perfect right because it would be an exercise in self-destruction.

The same thing holds true for anger—it's self-destructive. Cardiologist Ray H. Rosenman of the SRI International Research Institute maintains that angry people are more likely to die prematurely of all causes (including, presumably, diabetes) than their less hostile counterparts. Not only that, but chronically angry people fall victim to those irritating minor ailments like the flu and colds more frequently.

As a diabetic, a surge of anger can affect you like a piece of pecan pie, sending your blood sugar into orbit. (If you doubt this, take a test the next time you're in a perfect fury.) A quick and hot temper also doesn't make you a popular favorite with family and friends. Gaylen calls expressing anger "a form of public littering . . . how futile and dangerous it is." If you dump your emotional litter on everyone you come in contact with, you're likely to come in contact with fewer and fewer people as they go to great lengths to avoid you and your wrath.

How can you control your anger? It can be even harder than controlling your blood sugar. Maybe you have what David Burns calls a high IQ (Irritability Quotient) or what medieval physiologists would have diagnosed as a preponderance of black bile in your system; you're just naturally predisposed toward anger. Of course, diabetes can also induce a physiological anger. Low blood sugar can turn even a normally Merry Sunshine into a rampaging Godzilla. But even though it's not easy, you can learn to control your anger. Sometimes it takes innovative measures.

Dr. Gershon Lesser, in his book *Growing Younger,* told the story of one patient, a 47-year-old man with high blood pressure. As Dr. Lesser described him,

> He was the angriest man I had ever encountered. He did not wish to talk to me other than to say that he had been to five other doctors and none of them could cure his problem. I took his blood pressure and found it dangerously high, one of the highest I had seen in a man his age, and I had an intuition about what was killing him. The man was so abrasive, however, I dared not inquire beyond the most superficial of questions about his condition. I gave him some blood pressure pills, told him to cut out alcohol and cigarettes and put him on a salt-free diet and an exercise program.

Dr. Lesser's patient followed this advice compulsively, even making charts scheduling the exercise, pill-swallowing, and sodium intake. When his blood pressure stayed high, he returned to Dr. Lesser in a rage.

> His high blood pressure was now my fault, and it was rising to a new and extremely dangerous level. He screamed so violently that the other patients could hear him and were growing frightened.
> Finally, I dared to confront the man. I told him he was drowning in a sea of anger; that he needed psychotherapy or at least a punching bag on which to vent his anger, or he would die. Confrontation is not guaranteed to wake people up, but at the moment I felt it was his only hope. He stormed out of my office, threatening to sue me for malpractice.

The happy ending is that Dr. Lesser's confrontation got through the anger in this patient. He returned to the doctor's office a month later, a changed man.

He said that he'd taken a long look at himself and saw the sheer insanity of his wrath: mad at the world; punishing only himself. He said he drove to Sears, bought three punching bags (one for home, one for his office, a small one for his car). He said to me, "Go, ahead, Doc, take my blood pressure." I did. It was normal. "Those punching bags," he said, "they're better than your goddamn pills!"

Dr. Lesser agreed because, as he said, "all the medical knowledge and skill in the world cannot contend with the manifestations of the negative emotions."

Psychologist Albert Ellis, Ph.D., the founder of rational-emotive therapy, described another even more dramatic anger antidote in his book *How to Stubbornly Refuse to Make Yourself Miserable About Anything, Yes Anything!* One of his recovering anger patients helped stop his relapses by penalizing himself every time he got into a fistfight and every time he screamed at his wife. The penalty? He burned a hundred-dollar bill.

We'll now ask Dr. Rubin to explain how to keep yourself—and your hundred-dollar bills—from going up in smoke.

—June and Barbara

June and Barbara: In dealing with people with diabetes, the most common negative emotion we've found them expressing is anger. Some have even written us letters telling us how angry they are that our books don't have answers for one of their particular problems or complaints. We know of one young man, a dedicated fundraiser for the Juvenile Diabetes Foundation, who is now angry at that organization "because they haven't found a cure like they promised they would."

Whatever the cause, we can't help but feel that anger that is so pervasive and is nursed along year after year is extremely self-destructive. What is your experience in the anger arena, Dr. Rubin?

Dr. Rubin: Anger is an emotion most diabetics experience right from the start and continually from then on. When it comes to negative emotions, this is definitely one of the major ones. Dwelling on any negative belief is self-destructive, and when you refuse to let go of something you can't change, you're stuck, unable to move on, trapped in a futile effort to move the unmovable. Anger may be directed toward diabetes itself, all aspects of the regime, all persons involved in treatment, all persons who don't have diabetes, and even some persons who do.

Nursing your anger saps your strength so you have no energy left to make your life better. You may even believe that your diabetes makes a better life impossible. One woman told me, "I've had diabetes for 14 years, and I'm still angry. I can't achieve my goals because of my diabetes." Wrong! She couldn't achieve her goals because she had committed so much energy to staying angry.

It's *nursing* anger that's self-destructive. Feeling angry and moving on is not. In fact, acknowledging your anger is crucial to moving on. It's just that you can't stop there. It goes like this: "I'm angry, and I've got lots of good reasons to feel that way. Now what?" Hopefully, the "Now what?" takes you in the general direction of acceptance, healing, and making the most, rather than the least, of your life with diabetes.

June and Barbara: That makes beautiful sense to us. It's like the philosophy in *All I Need to Know I Learned from My Cat:* "Get mad when you're stepped on . . . Forget that you were stepped on."

Can you tell us some of the typical triggers for anger among diabetics and how people can prevent or neutralize them?

Dr. Rubin: The major trigger is the never-ending, unpleasant, nonnegotiable demands of life with diabetes. Many people experience these demands rather dramatically in terms of either imposition or deprivation. "Why me? It's not fair! Why didn't my sister get it? Why did my father have to give it to me?" "It makes me so mad that I have something I'll have to live with for the rest of my life!" "I can't stand the diet. Food is one of the few pleasures in my life and now they tell me

I'm supposed to eat like some kind of bird." "I hate shots! Sometimes I just feel like taking the syringe and throwing it against the wall. I'd rather die than turn into a pincushion." Some of this is natural, normal, inevitable, even healthy. So the first strategy is to accept these feelings. This acceptance can actually contribute to moving beyond resentment and anger.

If we consider health professionals as triggers for anger, I think a common feeling is that many of them do not really appreciate how difficult it can be to live with diabetes. Or maybe it's just that they do not communicate their appreciation. Here's what some of my patients say: "The doctors always make you feel like you're not doing good enough. That's really easy for them to say. They don't care about what you feel, and the way they talk, you know they don't have any idea how hard this all is." "The nutritionist gives you this diet that has nothing to do with real life. I'm working full-time, then cooking for my family, and she expects me to prepare another meal for myself. Right!" "The nurse asks me what I'm doing, then when I tell her the truth, she acts all offended, like I did something to her and she's mad at me. Where does she get off with that attitude?"

Another big trigger for anger is the feeling that many people who don't have diabetes tend to trivialize the demands of the regimen, while others assume the role of undesignated, uninvited, and unwelcome policepersons. "It really bugs me when I go to a party and see people stuffing their faces like there's no tomorrow, and I'm trying to be so good. They act so ignorant. What I wouldn't give for them to have my diabetes for just a little while." "People at work are always trying to tempt me with stuff I shouldn't eat. They always say things like, 'A little bit won't hurt you, will it?' It makes me want to kill!" Or maybe the problem is, "My family acts like they're prison guards and I'm the prisoner. They want to monitor my shots and my tests and everything else. Why can't they just mind their own damn business?" "My husband just won't accept the fact I've got diabetes. He expects me to do everything just as I used to, never takes my regimen or schedule into account. It makes me really resentful that he's so inconsiderate."

A pet peeve I hear from time to time is the tone in which some other diabetics talk about their disease. "The people I hate most are those diabetics who act like the whole thing is no problem at all. Where do they live, on another planet?"

Not to be forgotten as a source of angry feelings is extremes of blood sugar. I can't think of how many times I've heard stories about Dr. Jekylls turning into Mr. Hydes when their blood sugar skyrocketed or bottomed out. My son is a good example.

Eventually I could generally tell when Stefan's blood sugar was low just by looking at him. If I'd suggest he test his blood and got a response like, "I DON'T NEED TO!" I'd say, "You're right, you don't need to test your blood, go straight for the orange juice." My mild-mannered son got this way only when his blood sugars were low.

June and Barbara: You've certainly covered the gamut for anger responses. We could give examples from our experience of every one of these typical situations. So now we're all waiting to hear the strategies for preventing or neutralizing these anger attacks.

Dr. Rubin: First, accept the inevitability of these feelings. This alone will help you move beyond your usual outbursts of anger. The real issue here is how long they last and what you do with them when they arise.

Second, there is no satisfactory answer to the question of why you got diabetes and someone else did not. You're right, it's not fair. You have every right to be mad about that. You even have a right to stay mad for the rest of your life It's just not terribly smart to make that particular choice.

Third, treat the question of why you have to do what you have to do to take care of your diabetes (this is usually the foundation for feeling resentful and angry) as a real question rather than a rhetorical one. As a rhetorical question it just leads back to self-pity and anger. As a real question, it leads to looking at the choices you make for your life, health, and well-being. Be crystal clear about it: they are your choices.

No one, whether it's your spouse, best friend, or doctor, can tell you what to do or decide what's best for you. These are choices that only you can make. If you test your blood four times a day, it's because you choose to. If you eat sensibly, go to the doctor regularly, and exercise in a healthy manner, it's because you have made the commitment to these activities.

Similarly, if you decide to do none of these things, or if you make any choice in between, these are also commitments you have made. You may not think of it this way. You may think that your willpower, or your spouse, your boss, or your doctor, is responsible for what you do and don't do. But that's the old anger trough. The only way to avoid nursing resentment and anger is to truly accept the fact that *you* are continually making choices about how you want to live with diabetes. No one but you can assess these choices and their consequences.

Recognizing that you're always making choices can be liberating. If you don't like a choice you're making, you can make another one. Choosing to change some aspect of your life with diabetes is hard, but it sure beats the futility of waiting for someone else to make the change for you.

June and Barbara: You mentioned that some people's pet peeve is other diabetics who act as if diabetes is no real problem. We never realized until recently that we ourselves were sometimes causing this kind of reaction in diabetics. It seems that some who haven't gained good control feel resentful toward those who have. It's as if a person is thinking, "You're making me feel like a bad diabetic, because you're such a good diabetic."

June always thought she could help people most by proving by her own example that a diabetic can stay healthy and avoid complications with good care. She'd say to diabetics, "If I can do it, you can do it," thinking that she could inspire and motivate them. But with some, this does not work at all. How can people who react negatively to this message get rid of wasteful anger and resentment and use good diabetics as role models instead?

Dr. Rubin: I'll be the first to admit that there are a few diabetics whose attitude makes them a veritable magnet for resentment. They trumpet their terrific blood-sugar readings, or they talk as if it's a breeze to juggle all aspects of the regime with a full-time office job, a household with five children, and still have plenty of time to cook healthy, gourmet meals and for church activities, skydiving, and romantic weekends with their spouse. Their attitude may make it hard to resist throttling them or turning sharply on your heel and walking briskly in the opposite direction. But, wait a minute, maybe they've got something to offer.

If you see the "good" diabetic's success as a reflection of your failings, you're bound to feel resentful and angry. That's because your perspective determines your feelings. If you take a different perspective—that the "good" diabetic's success is a source of potentially useful information—then your feelings will be different.

How do you use other people's success, instead of railing against it? First, accept the fact that you're bound to feel both admiration and resentment. Don't waste energy fighting either emotion. Just because you admire someone doesn't mean you have to do everything that person does. And just because you resent someone doesn't mean you have nothing to learn from him or her. If you can accept your ambivalent feelings, you might be able to do yourself some good.

What is there to learn? Maybe a specific technique for making some aspect of your regime easier or more effective. Maybe a point of view that lightens your emotional load. Maybe a resource you could draw on. Or maybe this particular "good" diabetic has nothing to offer at all. (Hopefully, this will not turn you off to listening to others who may have some useful tricks up their sleeve.) If you see the "good" diabetic's behavior as a resource, not as a judgment on you, you can learn whatever there is to learn.

June and Barbara: Some psychologists point out that it's terribly detrimental to keep your emotions bottled up inside.

This seems to be particularly true of anger, which, they say, can fester within and create both physical and psychological problems. When we were working as college librarians, one employee was extremely hostile and often erupted in anger at the slightest provocation—and sometimes at no provocation. When she went into therapy for various other problems, the psychologist told her, "You mustn't keep your emotions bottled up," and urged her to let people know when she was upset about something. After that, she manifested even more anger and hostility. This created many problems for the library, since she was in a position in which she had to deal with the public.

During our years at the SugarFree Center, our hapless employees often found clients spewing anger all over them when they had done absolutely nothing to deserve it. After having been verbally beaten up for no reason by many furious clients, one of our employees sighed and said, "If I didn't know June and Pat and Ron [diabetic staff members], I'd think all diabetics were crazy."

In situations like this, we always tried to explain that the clients were not angry at the employee, they were simply displacing the anger they felt at having diabetes. As Gerald G. Jampolsky, M.D., said in his *Teach Only Love:* "I'm never upset for the reason I think." It seems that the greater the overreaction to a situation, the truer Jampolsky's statement is.

This is particularly well demonstrated in some of the letters received at the SugarFree Center. We remember one poignant exchange we had from a young girl.

June Biermann & Barbara Toohey:
Recently a concerned friend gave me a copy of your *Health-O-Gram*. I find it thoroughly disgusting and almost immoral that you are making money from diabetics. Diabetes is a serious illness and not a fun thing to live with for the rest of one's life. Why don't you fill your newsletter with helpful articles concerning good diabetic health care instead of making it into a money market?

I am specifically referring to the Injectomatic. You stated it enabled the diabetic to "get a pain-free shot of insulin every time." Well, I have news for you—there is no God-damn way to inject insulin painlessly. How dare you put hopes in my mind and countless others?

I am proud to say that I was one of the few smart people who looked into this device before sending you the $60. I called a diabetic clinic here in Milwaukee and they said it was a useless, expensive device.

I find it extremely sad and disheartening that you are making money on us. We have enough medical expenses without people like you trying to get more money out of us. I'd love to come to California and stick you with your Injectomatic and let you experience the pain and black and blue marks one gets from insulin injections. Then, possibly, if you are humane enough to understand my anger and disappointment in finding out this device is a piece of worthless junk, you will begin to realize how tragic it is that you take our hopes of painless injections and turn it into thousands of dollars for yourself.

Although we felt we understood the true source of her anger, this was an extremely disturbing letter to receive. We wrote to her that many people had, indeed, found that an automatic device helped them to give themselves painless shots, and we managed to finagle a free Injectomatic for her so she could find out for herself.

The next letter we received was a decided turnaround. She seemed to have had a personal epiphany. After apologizing for her outburst, she told us she had never truly accepted her diabetes, hated taking insulin (and consequently never mastered the skill of doing it correctly), hadn't taken good care of herself and was afraid she'd soon start developing complications. She told us she was determined to change. She was even considering working in diabetes education so she could help angry and rebellious young diabetics, because "I've been there and know what they're going through."

Some of our angry letters were so exaggerated that it was hard to take them seriously:

Dear Sirs [sic]:
I am enclosing my check for $2.50 to pay for the shipping of the book I ordered. Although you may not be particularly interested, I am dissatisfied with the book, which does not answer "All my Questions." I don't know if it answers any of my questions.

I don't doubt it answers all of someone's questions. It doesn't answer one question, however. Isn't $2.50 rather high for shipping one soft-cover book? I can answer that one myself. It certainly is, SugarFree people.

I eagerly look forward to never purchasing anything from you again, and I hope it is very soon.

We received the following note along with the return of a bottle of Lifesalt, a product containing 50 percent of the sodium of regular salt.

Gentlemen [sic]:
For the first (and last) time, I believed an ad.

If your people can honestly say this *crap* tastes like salt, please give them this bottle with my compliments. However, if they can't I would like a refund.

I have never tasted anything so bad; and for you to advertise that it tastes like common salt, is in my opinion, a crime. I couldn't get the bitter aftertaste out of my mouth with toothpaste and mouthwash.

Although many of us did use this salt ourselves, we gave the angry person a refund and a letter of apology. ("A soft answer turneth away wrath.")

When we received letters of this sort, we got some comfort from the fact that at least the person might have felt a little better after letting off some steam—steam that was undoubtedly generated by something other than what they were writing about. Probably that something was some aspect of their diabetes.

Even understanding that, it's still not pleasant to be on the receiving end of anger, so we were happy to read that not all therapists go along with the "for-good-mental-health-you've-got-to-let-fly-and-get-anger-out-of-your-system" theory. As we previously mentioned, psychoanalyst Willard Gaylen's theory is that, rather than blowing up, it's far better to resolve the situation that is the source of your anger. We have to counter, what if you can't resolve it or if the resolution takes a long time—maybe even years—or if you don't even know what the true source of your anger is?

Tell us, Dr. Rubin, what do you think about the virtues and vices of expressing anger?

Dr. Rubin: Venting your anger loudly and vociferously is one way of reacting to your feelings. Notice, I say *one* way. To my mind the vices of this way clearly outweigh the virtues. Think about the consequences of lashing out in anger:

1. Getting angry is physiologically detrimental to you. Anger triggers a fight-or-flight response that releases lots of adrenaline and other stress hormones. This can play havoc with your blood sugars and leave you emotionally wrung out.

2. The scene you create leaves both you and the person you attack miserable, and it takes a lot of work to resolve the hurt feelings.

3. Last of all, anger is so consuming an emotion that it completely distracts you from dealing effectively with whatever it was that triggered your anger in the first place.

Let's stop now and analyze anger as an emotion. It's a signal that something is wrong, that you're feeling vulnerable, scared, hurt, embarrassed, attacked, overwhelmed. This idea that anger isn't a primary feeling, that it's the result of other feelings, might not make much sense to you, and it's certainly not the way most of us see it most of the time. But bear with me. I'll bet that if you took any situation in which you felt angry and looked really closely at what you were feeling just before you got angry, you'd recognize that you were feeling one of the emotions I've just mentioned or another one that reflects vulnerability.

Let's say you were driving to work, for instance, and somebody in the next lane swerved in front of you, forcing you to maneuver frantically to maintain control. Naturally, you felt angry, but first, if only for a nanosecond (one-billionth of a second), you felt scared. How about another example? Maybe your doctor read you the riot act because your blood sugars were running high. You felt mad because he seemed so insensitive. My guess is that before you felt mad, you felt humiliated or guilty or both.

When you feel vulnerable—and this happens to most of us between 8 and 80 times a day—you can react in one of three ways:

1. You can react passively and simply bury your feelings.

2. You can react aggressively and lash out with anger.

3. You can respond assertively and deal with the situation straightforwardly.

Of the three choices, only the third works. If you stop to think about it, you can probably remember times you've been assertive. To be assertive means to give honest and direct expression to both positive and negative feelings in any situation. As Robert E. Alberti and Michael L. Emmons define assertiveness in their book *Stand Up, Speak Out, Talk Back* (Pocket Books, 1974), it is self-expression without stepping on others. Didn't it feel good to act in that manner? We all know people who seem to be consistently assertive. They speak their minds without getting angry, and they seem to get what they want most of the time, without pushing other people around.

If this isn't your general way of operating, you're not alone. Few people are consistently assertive. Why is this so, when the virtues of assertiveness are so clear and the vices of anger and passivity so obvious? First, and most important, few of us were brought up to be assertive. Instead, we were taught to be obedient. When we couldn't obey, for whatever reason, we got angry. Most of our early experience was in passivity and aggression, and old habits die hard, especially in the emotional realm.

June and Barbara: That explains a lot, even about ourselves. When feeling vulnerable or hurt, June is likely to become passive and Barbara angry. We guess that shows we're often still kids at heart—like most everyone else.

Dr. Rubin: Yes, it's as if someone were popping you into a time machine and transporting you back to some point in your childhood. You're left to deal with a crisis in the present with the emotional resources of a child. As children, you had only passivity and aggression to draw upon. You didn't have the resources to do anything but fight or give in. Now you do. As adults you can be assertive instead of settling for the untenable options of keeping quiet or lashing out.

June and Barbara: True, but that seems much easier said than done. How can we suddenly stop acting in a way to which we've become habituated?

Dr. Rubin: To become consistently assertive, you first have to recognize that vulnerability is triggering your anger. Then you have to recognize that you're probably reacting to this vulnerability instinctively rather than intelligently. Then you have to practice being assertive. I'll give you an example of assertiveness so you can see clearly the way it works.

Judy's husband, Dave, gives her the evil eye every time she eats more than she should. If she reacts by running out of the room in tears, she's responding passively and swallowing her anger. If she screams at him in a rage to mind his own business, she's acting aggressively. To be assertive, Judy could respond from a perspective of information-sharing. She might say, "You know, Dave, when you look at me that way it makes me feel awful, but it doesn't get me to eat less." Or, "I guess you think I'm overeating, but my blood sugar was a little low, and I think I need the extra bread." Or she might draw on her faith in Dave by saying, "I know I shouldn't have eaten that. And it's starting to feel like a pattern. Could you help me by telling me you worry about me when you see me starting to overeat and ask me not to do it for your sake? I think that might get to me."

Learning new ways to deal with anger is a lot of work. Each of the steps requires a lot of self-acceptance and patience. But it's well worthwhile because it could save your life. New research points to the direct role anger and other negative emotions have in coronary artery disease, one of the major complications of diabetes. I can also assure you that assertive living makes for a much more satisfying existence. Try it and see.

June and Barbara: On a radio call-in pop-psychology program, a woman with an eating disorder was told that when she stuffed down food she was really stuffing down the anger she felt toward the significant other in her life. The psychologist explained that she couldn't allow herself to give vent to her anger, because she was afraid it would damage her relationship. Have you ever heard this theory, and do you hold it yourself?

Dr. Rubin: Yes, I've heard it, and like most theories, it makes some sense. It fits with what I said about the sources of anger and the virtues and vices of expressing it. Stuffing food instead of expressing anger is a passive way of handling the vulnerability that is always behind anger. Of the three ways to handle anger, the passive response is anger turned inward, whereas the aggressive response is anger turned outward and the assertive response is active problem-solving. If you don't know how to be assertive (and most people don't) and you're afraid to be aggressive, you're left with only one option—turning your anger inward. Eating out of control is one way to do that. It's a form of self-punishment.

People with eating problems generally feel physically, mentally, and emotionally horrible before, during, and after their binges. Most people feel some basic, immediate gratification when they get a taste of something good, but the moment of pleasure passes quickly and the rest of the binge and its aftermath are generally pure hell.

Stuffing food to deal with basic vulnerabilities creates a self-reinforcing negative loop. By mistreating yourself, you confirm the fact that you aren't capable of anything better and that you don't deserve any better. You end up stuck in a cycle of self-abuse and self-hate. Not a pretty picture, is it?

If you have diabetes, the picture is even grimmer. First, stuffing food can wreck you physically. Lots of diabetics who eat this way end up skipping insulin to avoid gaining weight. This can lead to chronic hyperglycemia (high blood sugar) and its short-term problems and long-term complications. Other diabetics overtreat their binge-induced high blood sugars and end up with insulin reactions, which they also overtreat. Their blood sugars yo-yo up and down repeatedly.

The emotional consequences of overeating may be even worse than the physical ones. If there's one key to living successfully with diabetes, it's self-confidence. When you feel good about yourself, you can do what needs to be done. You can cope with the boring, demanding, frustrating, aggravating, and frightening moments that are part of daily life with diabetes. When you feel bad about yourself, this is impossible. You're running on empty, and you simply grind to a stop. You may even take a to-hell-with-it attitude. As one of my patients once said, "When you take a to-hell-with-it attitude, that's straight where you go."

Breaking this negative cycle is very difficult. When serious eating problems are part of the picture, it's usually impossible to resolve the issue without professional help. I'll talk more about that in chapter 10.

June and Barbara: In our experience we've found that the choice of words can create a lot of anger. For example, the word *cheating* is often thrown at diabetics by health professionals and even by themselves, as in "I shouldn't have cheated by eating that big cookie." When this word is used as an unjust accusation about a person's diabetes management, it causes anger.

Then there's the seemingly simple word, *diabetic*, used as a noun. When we first started writing and talking about diabetes, we always used the term *diabetic* when referring to people with the disease. Then we began to get irate letters objecting to this term. People would say things like, "I am not a diabetic and I don't want to be called one. I am an active, successful, complete person who just happens to have diabetes." Or, "There is one thing we all need to overcome: the reference to us as diabetics. I think this is stigmatizing, categorical, and inhuman. We are PWDs—people with diabetes—and not a separate category or genus." Or, *"Diabetic* is a label that sounds as if that's the only thing a person has going for him. I refuse to wear that label!"

This startled us and we were extremely upset at the idea that our innocent use of the word had so disturbed diabetics—correction, people with diabetes. Consequently, in our next diabetes book we went to all kinds of convoluted linguistic lengths not to use the dreaded word. It made for hard writing and equally hard reading.

When we were working on *The Diabetic Woman* with Dr. Lois Jovanovic-Peterson, we asked her opinion on this controversy. In the book, she replies, "Funny, I think the only people who are fussy about this are nondiabetics. I always say that it doesn't matter if I am a person with syphilis or if I am a syphilitic—I still have the same disease."

Finally, we decided that all this *diabetic* vs. *person with diabetes* stuff was ridiculous and started letting the word *diabetic* fall where it may in speech and in print. We have been doing so ever since, but we still occasionally get letters of objection, so it must be an issue.

What has been your experience with these two anger-trigger words, *cheating* and *diabetic?*

Dr. Rubin: Many diabetics describe those occasions when they stray from their diets as "cheating." This does sound judgmental to me, so I've never used the word. I've had similar, maybe stronger feelings about using the word *diabetic* as a noun to describe people with diabetes. This seems to define people by their disease. I made a habit of avoiding both these buzzwords. Then recently someone conducted a survey and found that most people with diabetes didn't mind calling themselves diabetics. Since then, I've asked lots of people how they feel about each of the buzzwords and found that a majority feel comfortable with both.

It all boils down to the meaning you attach to these words. If *cheating* and *diabetic* feel like simple descriptions without any negative connotations, use them by all means. If you feel otherwise, maybe we can come up with some alternatives. In place of *cheating,* how about *dietary indiscretion* (just kidding), *overeating, eating something I shouldn't have,* or *dietary noncompliance* or *nonadherence?* Actually, all of these sound judgmental, too. How about *grazing?* That's always been one of my favorites, though it really describes a particular form of cheating: nonstop nibbling. Maybe we should offer a prize to the person who comes up with the best alternative to *cheating.*

As for *diabetic,* the situation is more straightforward. You can use *diabetic person* or *person with diabetes.* That's more words, but, if you object to the naked *diabetic,* I can't think of any better choices.

➤ Help for Those Who Want to Help Diabetics

As we all know, diabetics (there we go again) can be very touchy about almost anything relating to diabetes and it's easy to push the wrong button and cause an emotional uproar. For example, few things make June angrier than being asked, "Do you have low blood sugar?" The question triggers anger, she says, because she's sick of hearing it; she's heard it around 3,587,062 times since she began using insulin. The question usually elicits the following response: "Do you think I have a little dial in my arm that registers my blood sugar? I have no idea if I have low blood sugar or not. Are you telling me to stop in the middle of what I'm doing and go test my blood sugar? Is that what you're saying?"

Barbara has been casting about for less wrath-inducing ways to put this question. The best one she's found is the one Richard K. Bernstein, M.D., offers in his book, *Diabetes Type II*. He suggests saying, "I'm worried that your blood sugar may be low. Please check it and let me know the result so that I'll feel less anxious." Surely no one could get angry at such a tender request. (Wanna bet?)

Do you have any general rules or specific cautions for family members and friends to help them avoid eliciting anger reactions from the diabetic in their lives?

Dr. Rubin: Here are Rubin's *Ten Commandments for Avoiding Negative Scenes with Diabetic Loved Ones:*

1. THOU SHALT NOT ACT LIKE A POLICEPERSON. This approach doesn't work and can ruin your relationship.

2. THOU SHALT NOT IGNORE DIABETES. Don't expect your loved one to carry on all activities as if the diabetes did not exist.

3. THOU SHALT NOT LEAD YOUR LOVED ONE IN THE PATHS OF TEMPTATION. Many diabetics find it upsetting to be constantly face-to-face with forbidden fruits, and they often get angry at the person who's eating those fruits in front of them.

4. THOU SHALT NOT CRITICIZE WHEN YOUR LOVED ONE SUCCUMBS TO TEMPTATION. Sure,

you're frustrated, but adding insult to injury is a surefire argument starter.

5. THOU SHALT NOT TALK ABOUT YOUR LOVED ONE'S DIABETES IN PUBLIC UNLESS INVITED TO DO SO. Public comments tend to be taken as criticism, so take your cue from your loved one.

6. THOU SHALT OFFER SUPPORT AND COMFORT, ESPECIALLY WHEN THINGS AREN'T GOING WELL WITH THE DIABETES. For any number of reasons, diabetics are often very touchy when their control is bad. A little extra TLC goes a long way toward avoiding confrontations at these times.

7. THOU SHALT HAVE THE PATIENCE OF A SAINT WHEN YOUR LOVED ONE IS ACUTELY HYPO- OR HYPERGLYCEMIC. These can be the worst of times, and if you both lose your heads . . . More on this issue later.

8. THOU SHALT DEAL CONSTRUCTIVELY WITH YOUR OWN NATURAL FEARS AND RESENTMENTS. Your diabetic loved one is not the only one living with the disease. You are, too, and you will feel scared, angry, even overwhelmed at times. You must find a way to deal with these feelings constructively, on your own and with your loved one. The key is to acknowledge what you're feeling and to take responsibility for the feeling. Some of the suggestions for doing this, made earlier in this chapter, might help.

9. THOU SHALT BE ESPECIALLY SENSITIVE IN PUBLIC SITUATIONS. Eating right, testing, and taking shots can be especially stressful for diabetics in public settings, so your diabetic loved one might be edgier than usual. Be alert for opportunities to make things a little easier.

10. THOU SHALT FIND OUT WHAT WORKS AND DO IT. In your family, a number of diabetes-related situations may often lead to conflict; for instance, when your loved

one has high blood sugar, eats something he or she shouldn't, or fights you when you want to help him or her deal with an insulin reaction. Find out what your loved one wants you to do in these situations, and do it. Don't wait until you're in the middle of a battle to ask, though. Ask when you're both feeling comfortable and relaxed. I never cease to be amazed at how well this simple approach works to avoid fights.

June and Barbara: This almost sounds like that song, "I was lookin' back to see if you were lookin' back to see if I was lookin' back to see if you were lookin' back at me." A diabetic gets low blood sugar and blows up for no good reason. The person who is blown-up at gets angry in return, which makes the diabetic even angrier, and this in turn makes the other person angrier still and on and on it goes.

Strangely enough, this happens even when the nondiabetic is experienced with insulin reactions. Not long ago we were setting off on a trip to New York. Barbara innocently asked if June had packed a recently purchased guide to the restaurants of New York. June exploded, "What a stupid time to ask if something is packed! Why didn't you ask about this yesterday? In the future you're going to be the one responsible for packing anything you want to take on a trip. I'm through getting blamed if something's missing!" She garnished these statements with a few expletives that have been deleted for family readership.

After picking up her dropped jaw, Barbara started ranting about what an outrageous way this was to behave when all she had asked was if the book had been packed. "I wasn't blaming you for anything. Why are you carrying on like this?"

June reentered the fray with fury. If the friend who was driving us to the airport hadn't arrived on the scene at that moment, it might have escalated into a screaming and shouting match, or worse. Barbara sulked off to load the car. June, to her credit, tested her blood sugar. (Actually, it was probably not so much to her credit as it was an automatic, habitual action because she might need to have a snack before leaving the house.) Her blood sugar was down to 33.

The funny thing is that after knowing June for the 25 years of her diabetes, it never entered Barbara's mind that June's aberrant behavior that morning would have anything to do with blood sugar. Funnier still was the fact that Barbara spent the whole morning "nursing her wrath to keep it warm," as Robert Burns put it. She kept muttering about how unfair June's outburst had been, even though she knew full well—and June kept reminding her—that it was not June but the low blood sugar that had started the whole thing.

How can a diabetic's family members and friends keep from reacting viscerally with anger when a diabetic is reacting hypoglycemically with anger?

Dr. Rubin: Your major mistake, Barbara, was that you failed to recognize June's attack as a symptom of low blood sugar. She really had you fooled. That's the first hurdle—to differentiate a reaction from the person's normal behavior. Always be suspicious of hypoglycemia when your diabetic loved one acts out of character or has a weird and sudden change of personality.

Even when you recognize these episodes, it's not at all easy to cope with them. A diabetic in the throes of an insulin reaction can be infuriating—argumentative, physically abusive, or simply outrageously irresponsible. One man told me that he started to scream at his wife in the middle of a round of golf they were playing when she offered him a glucose tablet. He was having a reaction and wouldn't admit it. Another man drank some orange juice his wife had brought him and then hurled the glass at her. One woman had a reaction at a mall 20 feet from several sources of food. She insisted in the loudest possible terms that she would not eat until she was taken home, a distance of ten miles.

Naturally, under these circumstances the support person feels unfairly attacked, unfairly burdened, or both. These feelings are totally justified. So what are you supposed to do? First, try to resist the temptation to beat your loved one about the head and shoulders or to walk away and abandon him or her to a well-deserved fate. At the moment you're the only one whose brain is functioning, so everything depends on you. To help you keep yourself on a fairly even emotional keel, try repeating to yourself this mantra: "This is not my _____ (fill in the blank with husband, wife, whatever). This is his/her evil hypoglycemic twin. In just a few minutes, if I don't add fuel to the fire, my loved one will return. In the meantime, I am not to take this personally."

June and Barbara: Aha! So the first rule is to keep your cool, and that's precisely what Barbara didn't do.

Dr. Rubin: Exactly. That's the whole secret. You're more likely to get a diabetic to accept treatment for the reaction if you remain calm. Remember what's going on: a reaction means the brain is starved for fuel. A starved brain operates irrationally. But even a starved, irrational brain responds better to a calm approach than to a frantic, frustrated one. I'm not promising you that the diabetic in your life will respond docilely. I'm simply saying that a calm approach works a lot better than the alternative. Even more important is personalizing your solution. Every diabetic I know responds best to some particular and familiar treatment. You need to work this out in advance. I was speaking to a group on this subject recently and got these responses:

> ➤ I always go along when my husband says, 'Do it for me.'"
> ➤ "My friend just holds out a roll of wintergreen mints and doesn't say a word. There's no fussing. I just take one."
> ➤ "I'm always willing to test my blood. If I'm low and my husband shows me the result without editorializing, I'll eat without fighting it."

As you can see, each person favored a different approach. All you need to do is figure out what works for you.

June and Barbara: What if people do get into a big emotional uproar? Are there ways to work your way out of it before it does real damage to the relationship? We've heard of cases where couples split up because of repeated hassles over blood-sugar reactions.

Dr. Rubin: One of the big problems with emotional scenes around reactions is that they tend to drag on, just as you suggest. People ruminate over some awful thing the other person said or did in the midst of the reaction. Or they blame each other for the fact that the reaction happened in the first place. Sometimes the fallout lingers for days.

Occasionally people stumble upon a wonderful air-clearing technique, which I recommend you try sometime. Many reactions have a humorous quality, ranging from absurd to macabre. I often hear people laugh about their reactions—usually well after the fact. Since you're going to laugh at your experience sooner or later, maybe it would be a good idea to make it sooner. The right time is once the low blood sugar has passed and before your mutual hurt feelings have had a chance to congeal into major resentment.

June and Barbara: Could you give us an example of how this works?

Dr. Rubin: Easily. A nurse I know is married to a diabetic man. Before going to bed one unusually warm night, they turned on a portable fan to pull in some of the cooler outdoor air. In the middle of the night the man woke up, told his wife he had to go to the bathroom, and got out of bed. Wondering why he had bothered her with this announcement, she noticed that he was staggering down the hall, not toward the bathroom but toward the room with the fan. Suspecting a reaction, she chased after him and arrived at the threshold of the room just in time to catch a faceful of fan-blown spray. She dragged her husband down to the kitchen and gave him his usual reaction antidote, orange juice and a few raisins. Then she mopped her face, thinking the worst was yet to come, because in the past her husband's reactions had sparked an escalating, acrimonious battle that usually took several days to run its course. This time she was in for a surprise. He started to laugh, louder and louder, until he almost rolled out of his chair and onto the floor. Totally taken aback, she asked what was so funny. "Just imagine," he sputtered, "what would have happened if I had been four inches closer to that fan!" She joined his laughter, and after a few minutes they wiped their eyes, hugged each other, and went back to bed. The reaction was over and the aftermath never materialized.

June and Barbara: That recalls to us the many occasions when June has done something so weird that years afterward we still laugh about it. One was the incident of the strawberries at breakfast, when June evidently ate her serving when her blood sugar was so low she couldn't remember doing so. As she came out of the reaction, she sobbed brokenheartedly and accused Barbara of having eaten the strawberries that she was so looking forward to. It took several minutes to convince her that Barbara had not purloined her strawberries. Then there was the time June started swearing like a sailor's parrot in our editor's office, but we won't go into that here.

We also know that high blood sugar as well as low can have an impact on a diabetic's personality. Let's tackle this problem here, too. Though less crucial than insulin reactions, high blood sugar can cause mood changes that other members of the family have to put up with.

Dr. Rubin: Yes, donnybrooks can be triggered by high blood sugar as well as low. One woman told me, "When I get high I feel like a witch sometimes. It's the ugliest feeling." A teenager said, "Highs make me feel sick and like I have no energy, which leads me to be moody and fight with my mother." An 86-year-old woman said, "My husband is always telling me I'm mean as a junkyard dog. But I think it's both of us."

Keeping your cool when your loved one's high blood sugars turn him or her mean calls for the same approaches suggested for dealing with low-blood-sugar-induced scenes. A diabetic is usually a little less irrational with a high, so it's easier to avoid a major hassle. On the other hand, highs tend to last longer, so you need to keep yourself together longer before your "real" loved one returns.

CHAPTER 4

➤

DEPRESSION
PITFALL

With our reputation for being almost pathologically happy, upbeat, fun-loving sorts, you can imagine how we were fretting
over trying to come up with an appropriate introduction to
this darkest of all emotions. Frankly, we were becoming somewhat depressed ourselves trying to get the right handle on
this heavy subject. Then, the benevolent and protective Universal Mind arranged for us to receive a perfect letter on the
subject. It was from Alan, a 28-year-old Southern California
filmmaker. He had been diagnosed diabetic only six months
previously and had seen our notice asking diabetics to get in
touch with us with any questions or experiences about the
emotional aspects of diabetes. This is what Alan wrote.

Dear Barbara and June:
As a relatively new diabetic who lapsed into a severe clinical
depression after my diagnosis, I think I might have some
thoughts and insights which could prove useful in your
research.
    Last summer I was directing a documentary in Hong Kong
when I began to lose a lot of weight. Since I had been very ill
on previous trips to Asia I didn't think too much of the weight

loss. What did concern me, however, was an increasing array of odd, disconcerting and downright painful sensations in my feet. Since there was no physical damage, I had a hard time convincing anybody that I wasn't imagining the sensations. I went to a series of doctors who gave me all sorts of orthopedic pads (which succeeded only in giving me all sorts of orthopedic problems—in addition to the increasingly weird and painful sensations), but nothing seemed to help. Because of my fear of drinking tainted water (which had sent me to a Bombay hospital a few years back), I decided to play it safe and drink lots of soft drinks. This was in addition to my steady diet of ice cream and Ho-Hos [a Hostess chocolate cake roll with creamy filling, the main ingredients of which are sugar, saturated fat, flour, corn syrup, eggs, and invert sugar] (I was so pleased that they had them in Hong Kong).

I was also working under a great deal of stress. I was racing to meet a schedule, I was desperately unhappy with the shape the film was taking and I was trying to juggle two other film projects which were collapsing around me. On top of this, I was staying in a small apartment where I was unable to get a good night's sleep because of the round-the-clock construction crew building a new high-rise next door.

Basically, everything that a person could possibly do to send blood sugar soaring, I did.

Needless to say, I was a wildly out-of-control diabetic. Although I had all of the classic symptoms, I was, unfortunately, not diabetes-savvy. Sadly, neither were the general practitioners I went to in Hong Kong and Tokyo. When I returned to the States, I met up with my parents in Florida. They took one look at me, set up an appointment with a local doctor and, sure enough, my blood sugar came in up around 800. I was hospitalized immediately.

That's when things turned really bad for me. Knowing essentially nothing about the disease (I was under the impression that I'd just have to cut back a bit on the ice cream and Ho-Hos), I was absolutely devastated as one horrific diabetic fact after another was dropped into my lap. I remember vividly shortly after the diagnosis picking up a copy of *Diabetes Forecast,* which someone had thoughtfully left for me. I flipped open to a letter from a lady insisting that diabetes was "a deadly killer" that "ravages the body" and that she was sick and tired of everyone being so upbeat about how easy it was to live with this incurable killer. Although she was making an argument in support of the new hard-hitting funding campaign, all I could think was "Deadly killer?! Ravages the body?!"

So far everyone had been so upbeat with me about how diabetes really wasn't so bad and that this diabetic person and that diabetic person lead perfectly normal lives and that great progress was being made in "management" of the disease . . . no one even hinted that my body was being "ravaged" by a "deadly killer."

When I started to look at the articles and ads in the magazine, I began to get a sense of what the lady was talking about . . . blindness, kidney failure, amputations, nerve disorders, heart attacks and on and on. It didn't take me long to figure out that this whole diabetes thing went way beyond ice cream and Ho-Hos. The last article in the magazine was a flippant, upbeat article by a diabetic woman who joked about losing her big toe (this little piggy went to market and never came back) because of her diabetes. This did not strike me as particularly funny. Then, as if on cue, a helpful nurse bounced into my room and cheerfully informed me that I had a hallmate who was also diabetic, and he was having both his feet amputated because of the disease. And so began my depression. . . .

Simple logic told me that if my sugars had been so high for so long (high enough, in fact, to have already given me one of the dreaded complications—neuropathy), then all the other dreaded complications must be just around the corner. All the pronouncements that if I kept good control blah, blah, blah . . . I wouldn't have to worry about complications, rang pretty hollow to me. I felt like I had never been given a chance to be in control.

Although I tried to be strong at first (I had seen so many movies of people overcoming adversities so much worse than mine), it wasn't long before I crashed. Aside from the constant discomfort of the neuropathy in my feet (and to make things worse, I now seemed to be losing feeling in my little toes, which I knew to be the precursor to amputations), I now had to deal with the petty daily annoyances of being a diabetic . . . sticking myself with needles twice a day, pricking my finger four times a day, not eating sweets (I had always had a voracious sweet tooth), eating absurdly small portions (4–5 cashews = one fat exchange!?), having my life regimented by my injection schedule (I couldn't sleep late because I would miss my morning injection, then I couldn't go back to sleep because I had to eat, then I couldn't take a nap because I had to exercise and so on). All this and what did I have to look forward to? Being a blind, bilateral amputee permanently attached to a kidney dialysis machine and in constant pain because of pervasive neuropathy. Life had become pretty bleak.

And it wasn't just the diabetes. As I slipped deeper and deeper into the depression, I grasped ahold of every aspect of my life that I had any dissatisfaction with and blew it wildly out of proportion. Anything I could blame on the diabetes, I did. And, of course, I blamed myself entirely for the diabetes. I tormented myself with an endless series of "what-if" and "if-only" loops. (What if I had applied for that great job in Hollywood instead of going to Hong Kong? If only I had come home earlier . . . If only I knew more about diabetes . . . Why did I drink all those goddamn soft drinks?) Not only was I convinced that I had no future to look forward to, as the depression deepened, I became increasingly convinced of the worthlessness of my past.

Things got worse and worse. The depression wreaked havoc with my sleep, especially in the mornings, which were particularly brutal. The less sleep I got, the more depressed I became. The more depressed I became, the worse my blood sugars. The worse my blood sugars, the more my neuropathy bothered me. The more my neuropathy bothered me, the worse my depression became. The deeper my depression, the angrier I became at myself for not handling the depression better, making me even more depressed, until I was eventually reduced to a near catatonic state.

My family, which had been blessed with a relatively problem-free existence, struggled desperately to deal with both my diabetes and, much trickier, my depression. A lot of mistakes were made on all fronts, but ultimately, through the loving persistence of family and friends, consultations with a psychiatrist (who was also diabetic) to whom my doctor referred me, the benevolence of time and an odd combination of jaunts to Trump Taj Mahal Casino and a Quaker retreat, I came out of the depression. In fact, my diabetes is now under excellent control, I have returned to L.A., where I'm writing and developing a variety of projects, and I am determined to do everything I can to stay healthy.

Although the neuropathy (for which I have not been able to find any relief, but with which I am learning to live) still occasionally gets me down, and though I am still fearful of what my period of severely high sugars may have done to my body, I am pretty good about shutting these things out of mind. Not surprisingly, as I get busier and more active, I find myself dwelling on these thoughts less and less.

Although I certainly do not look back fondly upon those hellish few months of depression and obviously would prefer not to be diabetic, I do genuinely believe that a lot of good has come out of the experience. My life is healthier and more balanced than it's ever been. I feel much better equipped to deal with whatever adversity, health-related or otherwise, may lay ahead for me. Finally (and I realize that this will sound a bit sappy and clichéd, but I really believe it to be true) I honestly believe that as a result of my diabetes and depression, I now have a little more insight, awareness, and appreciation of both the incredible suffering and incredible joy I see all around me.

During the six months since I was diagnosed, I have kept a detailed journal. As I reread it, a few things become evident: that depression is a serious disease which greatly distorts one's thinking (I am amazed at some of the things that went through my mind), that there really are a lot of day-to-day tangible things that can be done to "manage" depression while either the deeper roots of the depression are addressed or time begins to soften it, and that the depression wreaks havoc on one's physical well-being, especially if you have a chronic disease like diabetes.

I also recommend you read William Styron's book *Darkness Visible,* which accurately and eloquently describes much of what I and, I am learning, many other people have gone through.

Best regards,
Alan

We contacted Alan and he told us more about his depression and how he overcame it. He will speak to you again at appropriate places in this and other chapters.

—June and Barbara

June and Barbara: We hear a lot of diabetics say they're depressed. Could you explain to us what exactly a serious depression is and how you can tell whether you're just feeling down in the dumps or having a real emotional breakdown that you probably won't be able to get out of alone?

Dr. Rubin: A clinical depression, the official term for the real thing, is a treatable mental disorder. It's an exaggerated form of a normal emotional response to loss; in other words, an exaggerated sadness. Depression involves negative internal communication characterized by low self-esteem ("I'm worthless"), self-blame ("I can't do anything right"), and negative interpretation of experiences. Clinically depressed patients are particularly prone to make negative interpretations of situations when positive ones would seem to be more appropriate.

The symptoms of clinical depression are numerous. These are the leading signs that allow us to diagnose the problem: being bothered by things that don't usually bother you; poor appetite; feeling unable to shake off the blues; feeling inferior to other people; trouble concentrating; feeling that everything is an effort; feeling hopeless about the future; feeling your life has been a failure; feeling fearful; feeling restless; being less talkative than usual; feeling sad; crying spells; trouble falling or staying asleep; inability to get going.

When people talk about being depressed, they're rarely using the term in a clinical sense. They generally mean that they're feeling sad, blue, pessimistic, and at a low ebb in terms of energy. We all get down from time to time, but these normal downs come and go, unlike the state of clinical depression. I think of depression as the pits, the common lowest emotional state where all the other negative emotions settle if they aren't dealt with before they get completely out of control.

June and Barbara: We'd imagine that depression, either clinical or just symptomatic, would be more common among diabetics than nondiabetics. Is this true?

Dr. Rubin: A lot of research has been done on this question without a clear-cut answer. Different researchers come up with different findings because they study different people using different methods. One of the difficulties in assessing the incidence of depression among diabetics is the fact that some of the symptoms of depression coincide with some of the symptoms of high blood sugar, so when diabetics describe their symptoms, it's sometimes hard to tell whether they're depressed or hyperglycemic (or both). Recently, research has suggested that this confounding, as it's called, is not as great as we'd assumed, and that diagnosable clinical depression really is more common among diabetics.

June and Barbara: If we can't know for sure whether diabetics are more susceptible to depression, maybe you can at least tell us if there's any evidence that it is diabetes itself that causes clinical depression in those diabetics who develop it.

Dr. Rubin: It's almost certain that diabetes itself does not cause depression. Several studies, including one I carried out with my colleague Mark Peyrot at the Johns Hopkins Diabetes Center, indicate that the presence or severity of depressive symptoms is not related to the severity of diabetes, including the presence of complications. Other studies show that people don't consistently develop depression after they develop diabetes. Sometimes this happens, but the pattern can also be the opposite.

June and Barbara: Diabetes has to be related to depression in some way, otherwise so many diabetics wouldn't experience so much of it.

Dr. Rubin: Out-of-control diabetes does seem to be associated with an increased risk of depression. Chronic hyperglycemia, as indicated by elevated hemoglobin A_{1c}, is more common among diabetics who are depressed. This relationship may be the result of depressed diabetics taking poorer care of themselves, and this would result in higher hemoglobin A_{1c} levels. In one study, depressed and nondepressed diabetics were given blood-glucose memory meters and told to test their blood sugar. Though both groups did a pretty good job of sticking with the program at the outset, by the ninth week the depressed group was testing much less often.

Some scientists speculate that the relationship between depression and hyperglycemia may also be determined at a basic biochemical level. Similar changes in brain chemistry occur in the two conditions, and it may be that each condition potentiates the effect of the other. This means that the negative effect of depression on brain chemistry might make it easier for hyperglycemia to have its own similar negative effect (or vice versa). Or the negative effect of both these conditions together may be greater than the sum of each taken separately. That is to say, there may be a multiplier effect rather than an additive one.

June and Barbara: Aside from this biochemical relationship, don't high blood sugars bring on depression in psychological ways also? In their book *The Diabetes Self-Care Method,* Drs. Peterson and Jovanovic-Peterson point out that "high blood glucose over time . . . has an impact on mood."

Dr. Rubin: Yes, that's true, because people whose blood sugars are high often complain of mental and physical exhaustion, and this feeling of energy depletion activates a cycle that leads to depression. Let me show you how this works. I'll let two of my patients tell you about their exhaustion:

"I've always been a person in control, but for the past few years my diabetes has been controlling me. I come home from work exhausted, so I have to grab something fast and unhealthy to eat, which pushes my blood sugars way up, which makes me feel even more exhausted."

"I'm 68 years old and I've had diabetes for 28 years. I feel I've lost so much strength and health. Sometimes it seems that I just live in bed. I know part of it is depression and that I just need to push myself, but it's so hard to fight it."

So if a person believes that exhaustion is a sign of permanent decline or disability rather than a temporary and reversible state (as I might interpret my exhaustion after a 14-hour work day or a 20-mile run), he or she is likely to feel depressed.

Unfortunately, like most states of mind, both good and bad, the depressed state tends to be self-reinforcing: the more overwhelmed you feel, the less capable you are of taking care of yourself, and the less capable you are of taking care of yourself, the more overwhelmed you feel. The exhausted man who eats what he shouldn't and feels even worse is an example of this process.

I often have to make the point to people that feeling as if you have no energy and getting depressed about it are not results of diabetes per se, but rather of high blood sugars. I have to assure them that they're not over the hill because of their diabetes; that's just high blood sugars talking. And high blood sugars can be lowered.

June and Barbara: You know what we're going to ask next. What treatment can you give people to reverse the negative cycle that traps them?

Dr. Rubin: The approach I use for this problem is based on a cognitive-behavioral model. I believe that negative thoughts trigger negative feelings and that these feelings in turn trigger destructive behavior. The key to reversing the negative cycle is identifying and addressing the negative thoughts. This is an approach we've talked about earlier.

Cognitive-behavioral therapy has been proven successful in treating depression in nondiabetic patients. In fact, studies show that this treatment is more effective than antidepressant medication in terms of initial improvement and preventing relapses. I've adapted it for treating depressed diabetic patients.

June and Barbara: Can you give us an idea of how cognitive-behavioral therapy works?

Dr. Rubin: By way of example I'll tell you about a woman I treated recently. Evelyn has had diabetes for four years and was in a state of high denial most of that time. She refused to use the word *diabetes* to describe her condition, ate whatever and whenever she wanted, took her oral medication sporadically, and rarely kept appointments with her doctor. Not surprisingly, her blood sugars were almost always sky-high, so she was often exhausted, woke up many times each night to urinate, and had infections that she couldn't get rid of. She somehow managed to maintain her denial until she developed a particularly painful case of diabetic neuropathy (damage to the nerves). Her feet and legs felt as if electric shocks were passing through them, and they ached and ached.

The neuropathy, which struck about three months before she consulted me, devastated Evelyn. She had previously been very active. Now she had to go on leave from her job because she couldn't handle the standing and moving about it required. She spent most of her time lying in bed or on a couch in the living room, feeling like an invalid, shutting herself off from everyone but her immediate family and her parents. She was terribly depressed.

The silver lining of this tragedy was that it scared her straight. Evelyn finally accepted the fact she had diabetes and began to take care of herself. By the time I first saw her, her blood sugars were close to normal most of the time, she was taking insulin, testing her blood regularly, and attending diabetic support groups. But her neuropathy was no better, and she was still quite depressed. We began our work together by identifying the specific negative thoughts that were fueling her depression. (This was the cognitive part of the treatment.) Here are some of them:

> ➤ "My blood sugars are normal now. Why isn't the neuropathy better? Maybe it will never go away. I can't live like this."
> ➤ "I'm such a burden to my family. They are as supportive as they can be but it must be getting to them. When will they get sick of me?"
> ➤ "My family sits around talking and laughing sometimes, and I just want to scream at them for being happy. Isn't that awful? It makes me feel so guilty."

These thoughts and others in the same vein triggered deep feelings of futility, guilt, and rage. These feelings kept Evelyn from completing the process of healing, which she had begun when she started taking care of her diabetes.

June and Barbara: How did you go about helping her get rid of these negative thoughts?

Dr. Rubin: First, we talked about her neuropathy, trying to replace her self-defeating thoughts with ones that would reverse the cycle and create a mood where something good could happen. We talked about the fact that complications *follow* blood-sugar levels. The neuropathy she was suffering from was the result of the previous years of high blood sugars. Her current good control would be rewarded by relief from her symptoms, probably within a few months. That's how neuropathy works.

We talked about Evelyn's fear that she was a burden to her family, and she checked out this fear directly with them. She discovered that the real problem was not how much she depended on them, but her disappointment at no longer being the one upon whom everyone else depended. So she began to see that she was actually giving her family a chance to love her, that she was taking a kind of vacation (weird and involuntary as it was), and that she was having done for her what she had always done for others.

That's how we worked to replace Evelyn's negative thoughts with positive ones. The proof of the pudding for a positive thought is simple: it works for the particular person to create a mood where something good can happen. If a particular thought doesn't meet this test, we discard it and try another, until we find one that does work. The "something good" I refer to is a reversal of the downward spiral.

Now we come to the behavioral part of the treatment. Some of this behavioral improvement was already in place for Evelyn in the form of improved diabetes self-care, and some of it was bound to flow naturally from the positive thoughts and feelings we had triggered. But I believe in working on as many fronts as possible, and priming the behavior pump is almost always a good idea. After all, this is a cycle, so any improvement at any point in the cycle has benefits throughout the system.

June and Barbara: Why don't you show us how you primed this woman's behavioral pump so we can learn how to prime our own when the occasion calls for it?

Dr. Rubin: First you have to identify positive behaviors, and the place to start doing that is always with the person involved. Therefore, Evelyn and I made a list of things that already helped her feel less depressed. We started very simply, with things like getting out of bed at a certain time each morning, taking a shower, and getting dressed. We added buying a few new clothes, because Evelyn had lost a lot of weight. Clothes that fit well helped her feel better. Then she decided to start calling one friend a day to reestablish contact with the people she cared about and writing one thank-you note a day to people who had sent her cards and flowers. When it came to calls and thank-you's, the principle was, "A little at a time and the easiest one first." This helped build confidence. She also began taking daily rides with her mother or father, which they enjoyed.

As we listed the things that helped, we included some of the positive thoughts mentioned above. These thoughts included, "The neuropathy will get better in a few months if I just keep taking good care of myself." "This complication is the best thing that could have happened to me. Once I get better I can live a long, happy life." "I'm not a burden to my family. They love me and want to care for me." Evelyn kept this list in her pocketbook, and whenever she started to feel down, she would pull out her positive "menu" and choose something. Eventually whenever she seemed to be in a slump her family would say, "Get your list," and she would.

The work with thoughts and behaviors is directed toward creating the reality of *choices* where it had seemed before that there was only a grim future with no choice at all. After a few sessions, Evelyn told me she was over the worst of her depression. She had had a dream the night before that she was dancing, gliding smoothly in her husband's arms. When she awoke, her feet still hurt but she felt so much better emotionally that she knew she could manage until that, too, had passed.

June and Barbara: We weren't aware of the connection between depression and out-of-control diabetes. This brings up what we found out about depression in Martin Seligman's book, *Learned Optimism.* He indentifies the cause of depression as "the belief that your actions will be futile." Do you find that your diabetic patients who suffer from depression often believe that controlling diabetes is impossible?

Dr. Rubin: Just listen to a few of my patients on this subject:

"I've had diabetes for 18 years and it's getting worse all the time. My feet and eyes are going, and the doctors don't know anything to help me."

"I've had diabetes for 28 years. I've never been under control, and I've never been able to find anyone who could help me get under control."

"With my diabetes it's just one thing after another, from diet to pills to insulin. What's next? Do they cut off my feet?"

"I'm 34 years old and I've had diabetes 27 years. I've got bad complications, blocked arteries and kidney problems. I feel like I'm rapidly going downhill, and no matter what I do, nothing works. It's really discouraging."

"Do I have a pancreas without any beta cells or what? I feel like a leper and desperate for help. The problem becomes overwhelming at times. Somewhere in this vast world there must be someone to help."

Many people like those quoted above suffer from severe wear-and-tear responses to diabetes. This is not too surprising. As we've mentioned often, the regimen is demanding and unpleasant, and doing everything by the book doesn't always guarantee good results. Feeling different or damaged can sap motivation and lead to isolation, both of which add to the burden. What is common to all the demands of diabetes is the fact that they can leave a person feeling overwhelmed and convinced that all efforts are futile. A natural response to feeling overwhelmed is a to-hell-with-it attitude.

Throwing in the towel is the hallmark of depression. It's the sign I look for in my own work, the one that lets me know I'm dealing with a sure-enough depression. This attitude of futility is one element of a self-reinforcing, downward spiral that also includes destructive behavior (poor self-care) and negative physical consequences.

This spiral is likely to be particularly destructive if you're diabetic, because the spiral is usually steeper and harder to turn around when metabolic factors start interacting with emotional ones. In fact, there's evidence that depression is more malevolent (now there's a lovely term), more severe, and more likely to recur in diabetics than in nondiabetics. This means that depressed diabetics seriously need effective treatment.

June and Barbara: Would just normalizing blood sugars be enough to get people out of depression, or does almost everybody also need cognitive behavioral therapy?

Dr. Rubin: What you call normalizing blood sugars and I would call substantially improving them is a necessary but not always sufficient condition for resolving a depression. In some cases, improving glycemic control is all that's required. Feeling mentally and physically exhausted may be a temporary and highly reversible state related to nothing more than the level of blood sugars at the moment. Of course, this can be a pretty long moment if your blood sugars are generally out of control, but the point still applies. Try to get yourself to more normal blood sugars for a day or so, and see if your energy level doesn't rise and your perspective with it. If you can't get under control for even this long, to get a real sense of the "old you," at least try to remember a time when your control was better. Did you feel livelier? If you did, take my word for it that those days aren't gone forever. They're just buried under the high blood sugars, waiting to be retrieved.

This reminds me of what happened to my sister. She got an insulin pump about eight years ago and found that it improved her energy level and state of mind. She was amazed by this. She told me that even though her control had been pretty good in her pre-pump days, she would fall asleep on the couch each night after dinner. She was convinced that she was just "over the hill." Her control improved on the pump, and she suddenly found herself looking for people to meet and things to do every night after dinner.

But even dramatic improvements in blood-sugar control aren't always this effective in resolving depression. Evelyn, for example, found that her depression was still going strong even after her hemoglobin A_{1c} came down 50 percent, to a level that was almost normal. Though improved control was an important first step, she needed psychotherapy to get her fully back on track. For a little while I thought she might need an antidepressant drug as well.

June and Barbara: When do you recommend antidepressant drugs for diabetics?

Dr. Rubin: When I see a person who doesn't respond quickly and well to improved diabetic control and psychotherapy or a depressed diabetic who cannot achieve improved blood-sugar control, I consult a psychiatrist with whom I've worked closely for years. (A psychiatrist is an M.D. who can prescribe drugs, while a Ph.D. like myself cannot.) He sees my patient to determine whether an antidepressant might help. If this seems likely, he prescribes one and follows the patient to monitor the medication, while I continue the psychotherapy.

June and Barbara: What are some of the drugs you've found effective for diabetics?

Dr. Rubin: The antidepressant drugs we have used successfully fall into several different classes. First are the tricyclic antidepressants such as Elavil (generic name: amitriptyline), Tofranil (imipramine), Sinequan (doxepin), and Desyrel (trazodone). The most common side-effects of tricyclics include sedation, dry mouth, blurred vision, and constipation.

A second class of antidepressants are the monoamine oxidase (MAO) inhibitors, including Nardil (phenelzine) and Parnate (tranylcypromine). Patients taking MAO inhibitors must carefully watch their diet. Eating certain foods, especially fermented foods such as cheeses and alcoholic beverages, can lead to seriously elevated blood pressure.

Finally, there is the new antidepressant Prozac (fluoxetine). It is much more expensive than other antidepressants, but it seems to have fewer side-effects, especially sedative effects.

It is important to know that antidepressant drugs must be taken for several weeks before they are fully effective.

We use these drugs because they often relieve symptoms that reinforce the negative cycle. Once the patient is feeling more hopeful, energetic, and happy, by whatever means that state is achieved, it's usually easier to work in therapy and improve diabetes control. Remember, we're talking about cycles, positive and negative. We can intervene anywhere in the cycle and get it moving in a more positive direction.

Antidepressants probably work just as well for depressed diabetics as they do for depressed nondiabetics. I should mention that the effectiveness of all psychotropic (mood-altering) medications is an individual matter. Different medications, even those closely related chemically, seem to work differently for different people. Two things are important to keep in mind here. First, if you're depressed and seeking professional help, try to find a therapist who can prescribe medication or one who works closely with someone who can. Second, antidepressant medication should never be used as the sole approach for dealing with a psychological problem. It should always be used in conjunction with some type of counseling or psychotherapy.

June and Barbara: Do problems with diabetes ever cause people to go so far as to entertain thoughts of suicide? In all our years of working with people with diabetes, we've never heard of a single case of suicide.

Dr. Rubin: I know of no hard data on this issue. If the question is thoughts, not actions, then I guess almost everyone has thoughts of suicide at one time or another.

I've heard of only a few documented cases of suicide among diabetics. In a couple of instances the person took a massive insulin overdose; others used more conventional methods.

These numbers do not seem out of line with patterns among nondiabetics. Nor are my diabetic patients more likely than my nondiabetic ones to think or talk about taking their own lives.

But—and this is a big but—lots of my diabetic patients engage in a practice I call slow suicide. They're self-destructive when it comes to caring (or more accurately, not caring) for their diabetes. When I ask them what they think about their risk for long-term complications 20 or 30 years down the road, they often tell me they don't plan to live that long.

These folks talk as if they're planning to die before they have complications. So I ask what they have in mind, and almost always find the same thing: they have nothing in mind. They're simply feeling overwhelmed and helpless. They can't get themselves to do the right thing on the one hand, and they can't face the consequences of doing the wrong thing on the other, so they generate a magical, if decidedly morbid, solution to their dilemma: they'll go on as they are, and then somehow check out before they confront the fate that awaits them. People in this boat rarely commit active suicide, but unless they see the light, they may end up achieving the same result more slowly.

June and Barbara: Since we're great advocates of exercise, we always mention in our books that it's good for raising the spirits as well as lowering the blood sugar. We've had reports that it really works. For example, our pen pal filmmaker, Alan, told us that he found that diving into cold water and swimming laps or getting a cold jolt of air riding his bicycle helped him when he was in his depression. He said it made him feel really alive. He also said he got that same kind of rush of excitement and alive feeling when he gambled. (That was how the Trump Taj Mahal Casino fit into his coming-out-of-depression story.)

We won't ask you to suggest that diabetics should take up an activity like gambling, which many people consider sordid and immoral and others find addictive, but how about exercise? Could you recommend that as a way out of depression or at least a temporary respite from it?

Dr. Rubin: Yes, yes, a thousand times yes. Exercise is wonderful, whether or not you have diabetes and whether or not you're depressed. It's a veritable fountain of well-being. If you're depressed and diabetic, drinking from this fountain can be especially beneficial.

First of all, exercise can improve your blood-sugar control, just like *that*. I've seen my son's blood-sugar level go from 240 mg/dl (13.3 mmol/L) to 80 mg/dl (4.4 mmol/L) within 45 minutes when he's really active. Exercise is also an essential element of a sensible weight-loss program. So Type II's can often generate long-term improvements in their control if they really get into exercise. We've already talked about the importance of avoiding hyperglycemia in the treatment of depression.

Exercise also seems to activate those magical brain chemicals called endorphins that give runners their high. People who exercise regularly know and love the feeling they get from these little guys. Whether or not you believe in these neurochemical wonders, there's no denying the fact that regular exercise improves your self-esteem and self-confidence. If you're fighting depression, these benefits are like gold. When you walk, run, bike, skate, swim, dance, or ski regularly, the exercise improves your appearance. Even more important, your exercise accomplishments provide a crucial depression-banishing lesson: YOU CAN DO IT. In response to my earlier comment that the essence of depression is a state of mind characterized by feelings of futility, your exercise successes can be a powerful object lesson to the contrary.

As you may have surmised, I use exercise to foster my own self-confidence. I run a lot, and most times during the first mile I consider stopping. Maybe I'll have a little ache (this does tend to happen in middle age), or I'll remember something else I could or should be doing. When this feeling hits me, I remind myself that I've run about 5,000 times in the last 15 years and I've had this feeling approximately 4,000 of those times. I've almost always carried on despite the feeling. And on about 3,990 of those 4,000 occasions, the feeling has passed quickly and I've completed my 5 or 10 or 15 miles comfortably and happily. I apply this lesson to other aspects of life all the time. I'm often faced with situations where I'm tempted to give up. I try to do the same thing I do when I run—have confidence and persevere. This attitude and the behavior it generates tend to create a positive self-fulfilling prophecy, the perfect preventive (or antidote) for depression.

That's not all. Exercise is relaxing; it's a great way to work off physical tension and some of the anger you might feel when you're depressed. It's also a wonderful opportunity to think. You get a nice, healthy flow of oxygen to your brain so that it operates at high capacity. Clear thinking is a must for working through a depression and assuring it doesn't return.

So do yourself a favor, exercise. It doesn't have to be anything major at first. In fact, it shouldn't be. Start very easy, with something you like, at a level you know you'll find comfortable. Even walking one block can be the beginning of something wonderful, if you stick with it and build up as your capacity grows. Just figure out what works for you. Do you like solitary exercise, or would you prefer to join a club? Are you already in pretty good shape, or are you starting from square one? What are the easiest times for you to work out? As little as 30 minutes three times a week will make a real difference.

June and Barbara: We're just as gung-ho for exercise as you are. In fact, in our advanced years we've joined a new gym in our neighborhood. We'd read that muscle-strengthening exercises are just as important as aerobic exercise, and though we were walking about four miles a day, we were neglecting this other aspect of keeping in good condition. June in particular was hesitant to try the muscle-building machines, because she has a bum left knee from a bike fall and a plastic thumb joint in her left hand. She overcame her fears (negative thoughts), signed up, and finds that her knee and left hand and arm have improved from using the equipment instead of the opposite. Think what a mental lift that gives a person! Another important plus is the time-saving factor. In one hour we can get in

20 minutes of aerobic training on the gym's exercycles and 40 minutes of muscle strengthening. As you say, it's a question of designing your exercise program to fit into your schedule so you can do it regularly. As Alan says, "You have to make it a part of the weave of your life."

If you get really serious about exercise, you might want to join the International Diabetic Athletes Association. This is a nonprofit organization formed in 1985 to foster interaction among individuals with diabetes about the risks and benefits of exercise. The group has a newsletter and active chapters in different cities. To join, write them at 1931 E. Rovey Ave., Phoenix, AZ 85016, or call 1-602-230-8155. Dues are $12.00 a year.

Among the hundreds of diabetics and their family members and friends we've talked with, however, we've noticed something we've come to call the "yes, but" syndrome. Here's how it goes. Someone has a problem, so we suggest something that will help resolve it. The person acknowledges that this is a good idea, and then follows up with reasons why he or she can't possibly do it. An example might help you get the idea:

We: If you would get on a regular exercise program, it would help keep your blood sugars normal, help you lose weight, and just plain make you feel good."
They: Yes, but I don't have time.

We: You could get up an hour earlier in the morning and exercise then.
They: Yes, but I already have to get up early to fix my special breakfast and get the kids off to school. I couldn't do it then.

We: Okay, then you could take a walk during your lunch hour.
They: Yes, but there are always so many crises at work, I can hardly get away from my desk at all. Anyway, I don't want to get all sweaty and windblown. There's no place to

clean up at work and I have to keep up my appearance in front of the clients.

We: Well, you could always exercise in the evening after dinner.
They: Yes, but it's too dangerous on the streets at night. I couldn't go out then.

We: You could join a gym and work out there.
They: Yes, but there isn't a gym near where I live. It would take too long to drive to one.

We: You could get an exercycle or a rowing machine.
They: Yes, but I have no place to keep one.

We: You can slip a rowing machine under your bed or the sofa.
They: Yes, but they're too expensive. I can't afford one.

We: Well, then you could just get a few feet of clothes-line and jump rope in the evening. That would cost almost nothing and would be easy to store.
They: Yes, but I live on the second floor of an apartment and my neighbors downstairs would never put up with me thumping on the floor every night.

And so it goes. People who are victims of this syndrome have a "yes, but" for everything. What causes people to acquire this syndrome, and what can they do to get rid of it when, especially if they're depressed, it is so difficult for them to change their thinking or their actions and reverse the downward spiral?

Dr. Rubin: The "yes, but" syndrome is simply depression by another name. It's a clear sign that the "yes, but-er" is overwhelmed and feels that any action in the service of improved diabetes self-care is doomed to failure. You're right that no positive change is possible while the victim of the syndrome remains in its grip.

I think we've already covered the approaches that might be effective. I might start by trying to identify the underlying structure of attitudes and beliefs upon which the "yes, but-ing" rests. After hearing a series of suggestions rejected, for instance, I might say, "I've offered lots of ideas for getting started with the exercise program you say you want, and none seems workable. Can you think of anything that might work better than the suggestions I've made? Maybe my ideas stimulated your thinking." If the answer is yes, we have something to work with.

June and Barbara: What if the answer is no—as it often would be?

Dr. Rubin: If the answer is no, I'll say, "Hmmm, so *nothing* could work. I wonder why."

The response to this might be, "I just don't have the time" (or the energy, or whatever). This is the point where I try to introduce the notion of a choice. If the issue is time, for instance, I'll note the things the person does find time to do (watch television, read magazines, visit friends). Then I'll say, "So it sounds as if you're choosing TV, reading, and visiting friends over exercise." I try to avoid sounding judgmental; I'm simply making an observation. If my comment is taken as a judgment, I do my best to correct that misperception. That's very important, because treating my comment as a judgment creates a confrontation (active or passive) that diverts our attention from the real issue. It isn't easy to avoid this trap, and it's also not easy to help a person see that choices are being made when other activities happen and exercise doesn't. But I've found that I can often help the person make this crucial step toward freedom from "yes, but-ing" if I gently stick with it, repeating over and over again that I'm simply making an observation, not a judgment.

June and Barbara: Why is it so important for the person to accept the idea that he or she is making a choice?

Dr. Rubin: Because this gives the person power—most importantly, the power to change. Once you see your behavior as a choice, you're no longer stuck with the old feeling of hopelessness and futility that is the foundation of the "yes, but" syndrome. Now you must say one of two things: either, "Yes, I do make the choice to put a low priority on my exercise," or "No, I don't want to continue making that choice, I'm going to find a way to make exercise a priority."

Even if you choose to place a low priority on exercise, you've still taken an important step, because you've placed your behavior in the context of a *won't* rather than a *can't*. That opens the door for further thought and a possible reordering of your priorities some time in the future. If you accept that not exercising is a choice, you're also accepting that you can change your mind and make a different choice. You're empowering yourself. If you decide right away to make the choice to exercise, so much the better. You can begin to think of ways to put your choice into action. You'll need to do two things. First, shift some of your energy from other priorities to exercise; and second, start your exercise program in a way that maximizes your chances of succeeding at it. I offered some hints for doing this in my answer to the last question.

Any way you cut it, recognizing and acknowledging that you're making choices is the way to cure the "yes, but" syndrome.

➤ Help for Those Who Want to Help Diabetics

Our friend Alan, who chronicled his depression for us in the letter at the beginning of this chapter, made some important points when we talked to him later. He was adamant that a depressed person should never go to the diabetes doctor alone.

A friend or family member should go along and sit in on the discussion.

Alan's reason for this recommendation, based on his own experience, is that the depressed person will only remember the negative things he hears from the doctor. The positives all flow right through his ears without making a brain-stop. He will also remember the negatives he was told as being far worse and more insurmountable than they actually were. The person who was with him will need to constantly remind him of things that were said that could give him a more optimistic outlook.

Another thing that helped Alan out of his depression, he said, was that "my friends would come by every day whether I wanted them to or not. Thank God!" The depressed diabetic may flatly tell you he doesn't want to see anybody or do anything with others, when doing something with somebody is exactly what he needs.

Barbara had a friend who was depressed in recent years, and all she could think of doing for her was taking her out to dinner and talking with her. June used to make fun of Barbara's efforts, saying, "She's in a state of clinical depression. What possible good is taking her out to dinner going to do?" The things that Alan said about his friends make Barbara feel somewhat vindicated in her administering of dinner therapy. At least, she got her friend out of the house and moving.

Dr. Rubin, what do you think of dinner therapy or walk therapy and other such friend-administered unscientific treatments?

Dr. Rubin: I think of friends as life jackets for a person adrift in the Sea of Depression. Their steadfastness, love, and support are an antidote to the poisonously negative world view that is the hallmark of depression.

When people are depressed they believe they are worthless, that life is not worth living, and that the future is hopeless. Think about how your friendship can help when a person is feeling that way. You lovingly hang in there, and that's bound to have some effect on your friend's self-esteem, day-to-day quality of life, and hopes for the future.

So yes, I support all manner of friend-administered treatment for depression—with one caveat. The treatment has to be steady and dependable to be effective. Given the depressed person's proclivity for negative interpretations, inconsistent support can create real problems; it may even backfire, convincing the depressed loved one that no one can be trusted. So when you're providing support, pace yourself for the long haul. This is really important because depression can go on for months, and you will likely feel very drained staying supportive that long. One woman described her depressed friend as a black hole, sucking energy from everyone who got close to her and giving back almost nothing.

When providing support you also need to remember what you can do and what you can't. You *can* be a life jacket, helping your friend stay afloat. You *can't* be a motor, providing the impetus to carry him or her back to dry land and freedom from depression. This your friend must do alone, or with professional help, if necessary.

June and Barbara: People have a tendency to want to get the depressed person to cheer up and get over the bad feelings right away. Alan considers it inappropriate to start trying to cheer someone up immediately; he thinks the person needs to have time to mourn the loss of the things that have to be given up. It's hard not to try to cheer up the depressed person when you see him so down, but is it wrong or at best counterproductive? If you aren't supposed to try to cheer up your loved one, what *are* you supposed to do?

Dr. Rubin: This relates closely to the previous question. When you try to cheer up a depressed friend, your efforts are likely to backfire. Rather than feeling supported, your depressed friend or loved one is likely to think you don't appreciate the depth of his or her pain—and of course you don't. In fact, you can't. Your cheer-up noises often leave your loved one feeling even more isolated and depressed.

I'll be the first to admit that the temptation to cheer up a depressed person is almost irresistible. After all, the person's negative views are obviously out of touch with reality. (That's what being depressed is all about.) Plus, it's a drain to be with a friend or loved one who has sunk so low as to become a "black hole." So, your cheering-up efforts are an attempt to maintain your own balance, too. But cheering up is futile, or worse, unless you are invited to do so. Even then, try not to come on too fast or too strong.

June and Barbara: What are you supposed to do if you feel you want to do *something* to help?

Dr. Rubin: You might try to help your depressed loved one identify the particular negative beliefs that are fueling the depression. But this is a very delicate task. It's easy to slip over into trying to counter these beliefs yourself, and that almost never works. You could help your loved one see that this is probably a full-fledged depression, if that's how it looks to you, and suggest professional help. But most important of all, try to be there in the ways I have suggested. Help keep your loved one afloat while he or she finds the strength to strike out for shore.

GRIEF
GOOD GRIEF

When people are diagnosed as diabetic, many have a grief response that is not unlike the one experienced at the death of a loved one. This isn't surprising since they are experiencing many kinds of death: death of life as they knew it, death of freedom, and death—or at least curtailment—of some of their most cherished activities.

An even more significant passing is the passing of the idea all of us secretly harbor—no matter how intelligent or realistic we may otherwise be—that we're invulnerable and immortal. "Sickness and death happen to other people, not to me. A world without me is unthinkable." Suddenly, thanks to diabetes, you start thinking the unthinkable and grieving this inevitable and profound loss of self.

We said earlier that none of these so-called bad emotions is all bad. They serve a useful purpose. This may hold more true of grief than of any of the others. As the poet William Cowper said, "Grief is of itself a medicine." However bitter it may be, we need to swallow it, let it do its healing work, and get on with a new life, a life that can be more meaningful to ourselves and others than the previous, less aware one was.

As the playwright Edward Albee said, "All of my plays are about people missing the boat, closing down too young, coming to the end of their lives with regret at things not done, as opposed to things done. I find that most people spend too much time living as if they're never going to die. They skid though their lives. Sleep through them sometimes."

When choreographer and Joffrey Ballet star Edward Stierle was diagnosed as having AIDS, he told a *Los Angeles Times* reporter, "It changed my life dramatically, but it didn't ruin it. I didn't just crumble. In actuality, I started living more." He even referred to his diagnosis as a wake-up call that forced him to redirect his life. Soon after his diagnosis he created his most acclaimed ballet, "Lachrymosa."

June never had this kind of conscious reaction to diabetes. She never said to others—or even to herself—that it made her want to do more, to redirect her life, to make dramatic changes. But somehow, after diabetes, she found herself doing more in both work and play, making radical career alterations, and embracing change in all areas of her life, often quoting the Buddha: "The only constant is change."

She also became more careful with the hours and days of her life. Since she no longer felt she had an unlimited bank account of time, she no longer squandered it. Instead she spent what time she had judiciously, making sure she always got top value. (And, as her friends learned to their chagrin, she became monumentally intolerant of time wastrels, no matter whether they were throwing away their time or hers, or, more likely, both.)

But before you can make your own positive life-enhancing changes, you have to first work through your grief. You can't just ignore it or suppress it. "Suppressed grief suffocates," said Ovid. It also won't stay suppressed. It will pop out later on down the line, stronger and more difficult to cope with than ever.

We'll now ask Dr. Rubin to help you understand, accept, and deal with your grief so you can emerge from it whole and uncrumbled and use it as a wake-up call, a springboard into a new, better, more exciting, and worthwhile life.

—June and Barbara

June and Barbara: Despite the fact that diabetes is not a terminal illness, we've read many articles that explain that when you're diagnosed diabetic, you're likely to experience a grief response that takes you through the stages that Elisabeth Kübler-Ross describes in *On Death and Dying*. These stages are: denial, anger, bargaining for more time, depression, and, finally, acceptance. Does the grieving process in diabetes follow the same pattern as that of terminal illness?

Dr. Rubin: The stages of adapting to a terminal illness do apply to diabetes, but what Kübler-Ross described is a model of the grieving process. A model is an abstraction; it oversimplifies in order to highlight important facts. It's true that most people adapting to diabetes have most of the feelings Kübler-Ross identified. It's also true that these feelings are usually first experienced in the order of Kübler-Ross's stages. But it's not true that most people move through the grieving process smoothly from stage to stage: denying, then feeling angry, then feeling depressed, and so on. People tend to go back and forth among these stages, day to day, and even minute to minute, as their lives with the disease unfold. Many people even feel they are in two or more stages at the same time.

So, the actual process of grieving diabetes is almost always "messier" than Kübler-Ross's model, and for some people it's particularly messy. Some get stuck in one of the stages: denial or depression, for instance. Others move back and forth between anger and depression. The rest of this chapter is devoted to figuring out why grieving and healing are so hard for some people and how to make the process easier.

June and Barbara: Even though few diabetics make an unwavering, straight-line march through the Kübler-Ross steps, could you give us a paradigm of how the grieving process goes from diagnosis to acceptance?

Dr. Rubin: As you mentioned, many people react to a diagnosis of diabetes as if some important part of them had died. One man told me that he felt like his life ended the day he was diagnosed. Others mourn a loss of self-confidence, of spontaneity, or of things they love to do like golfing, camping, or cutting wood. Still others say that having diabetes makes them feel like invalids or second-class citizens.

People grieve when they must face the loss of something they value, whether it's a job, a beloved pet, a marriage, a life without diabetes, or even life itself. The grieving process that Kübler-Ross identified in people with terminal illnesses applies to any loss. Since the losses we're talking about can't be reversed, the goal of healthy grieving is acceptance. Each stage of grieving has its place in the process.

Denial or shock is a natural first reaction to a diagnosis of diabetes or terminal illness. As I pointed out in the denial chapter, this is actually a healthy reaction, because denial protects us from emotional overload.

After a while, the reality of the diagnosis begins to sink in, and the second stage of grieving—anger—follows naturally. Having diabetes (or facing death) is terribly unfair, so you're bound to feel angry. Anger is a healthy response at this stage, just as denial is at the outset.

Bargaining for more time is common in terminal illness, because you haven't died yet when you're diagnosed. It's much less common with diabetes, because you already have the condition. I have, however, seen this kind of bargaining in some people with Type II who may work on their weight to avoid oral medication or work with oral medication to avoid insulin.

When the full impact of loss settles, depression often follows. In the months following a diagnosis of diabetes, many people go through a period when they feel hopeless, helpless, and overwhelmed. Once again, the feelings are natural, if not inevitable. So much has changed. As one man said to me, "Six months ago, before the diabetes, I had the world. Now I've lost it."

Grieving is an ongoing process of emotional healing. The ultimate goal of grieving is acceptance. Acceptance means dealing with the reality of diabetes in the context of a life that feels whole again.

June and Barbara: Does the way the significant people in your life treat you after your diagnosis affect your progress through the grieving process—speeding it up, slowing it down, making it easier, making it more difficult, or even stopping it dead in its tracks?

Dr. Rubin: Absolutely. When people are really there for you, the grieving process is much easier. Being there for you means putting you first at this crucial time. It means loving you, listening to you, and finding out what it is that you want and need. This is a tall order. Really being there can be difficult even under normal circumstances, and these aren't normal circumstances. Your family and friends are going through their own grieving process. Unfortunately, many family members and friends get hung up on their own agendas, and this can make your grieving process harder.

Some people respond to a loved one's diabetes in a way that gives the diabetic little room to grieve. A young woman I know drove home from college to tell her parents of her diagnosis. She found her father sitting at the kitchen table, eating ice cream. She blurted out her news. Never looking up from his bowl, her father responded, "Just be thankful it's not cancer." Ouch!

Other people tend to overwhelm the diabetic with good cheer, immediately citing every advance in diabetic technology they can bring to mind. Certainly, there are many things worse than a diagnosis of diabetes, but that's a realization *you* must arrive at, *after* you've done whatever grieving you need to do. People who want to transport you there instantaneously are actually delaying your journey, not facilitating it.

June and Barbara: Humor is not common at this time, but June still cherishes a postcard sent to her by a Los Angeles Valley College colleague shortly after her diagnosis. "My aunt had what you have," he wrote, "and she lingered and lingered." This made June laugh out loud—which is always good therapy—and it effectively straddled the line between having people make light of a situation, which is bad, and acting as if your world has come to an end, which is worse.

Dr. Rubin: An even more grief-hindering response is when people approach you with long faces, hand-wringing, wailing, and a litany of sad stories, told in hushed voices, about their great uncle who lost both his legs and then died of kidney failure. They treat you as if you were already halfway to that state yourself, as if diabetes were a terminal illness.

Some close family members may take a different tack. They get so upset about how your diabetes affects them that they completely lose sight of the fact that *you're* the one with the disease.

All the unsupportive responses I've described flow from the same source: fear. People tell you that you have nothing to worry about, or everything to worry about, or that *they* have everything to worry about, because they're scared. They're so scared that they can't be there for you. Unfortunately, this is a time when you really need support, so these responses can make it harder for you to grieve and heal.

June and Barbara: One thing diabetics virtually universally grieve over is the loss of freedom of food choices. We've heard people mourning over the doughnuts or pecan pies of yesteryear. Children mourn the loss of all sweets. Men often recall with nostalgic longing the good old days of drinking multiple beers with buddies. Consider June's dismal "last supper" on the day of her diagnosis. Just how do people console themselves over all these "I can't have anymore's" or "I can't have as much as I used to's" that diabetes imposes on their diets?

Dr. Rubin: Food deprivations are probably the single most common source of grief among diabetics. I've heard people say things like, "Food is my strength," or "I live to eat," or "Giving up all those goodies makes me feel like I'm losing my best friend." Food is that big a deal for many people. Food is not just a way to stay healthy; it's a source of emotional comfort, a way of giving and receiving love, and a major focus for many social activities. It's no wonder food restrictions are often so painful.

One man really brought this home for me with his story about a Thanksgiving dinner. His mother had died recently, and he was sharing the holiday with both of his sisters for the first time in 20 years. The repast included many special dishes his mother had prepared on previous Thanksgivings, so the meal had many aspects of a ritual. Yet the man felt left out because he couldn't partake as freely as his sisters.

How do you console yourself under these circumstances? The key is to avoid feeling overwhelmingly deprived, and the man I've just described found one way to do this. He told me that despite his disappointment, he felt good about himself because he was able to stick to his diet even under pressure. You deserve to feel good about yourself when you do the right thing, because doing the right thing can be so damned hard.

Another way to avoid feeling overwhelmed is to let yourself get angry, as long as you are just blowing off steam. Stewing in your anger, on the other hand, generally hurts more than it helps.

Still another way to avoid feeling overwhelmingly deprived is to enjoy—in fantasy—those things you're not supposed to eat. This probably sounds strange, but you might want to give it a try. Think of your favorite forbidden fruit. Maybe it's a particular ice cream or candy bar, or maybe it's fried chicken. Picture yourself eating as much of this wonderful no-no as you want. Taste the luscious flavor of the ice cream, feel the coolness in your mouth, the crunchiness of the chocolate bits and nuts. Mmmmmm! The risk here is that your fantasy may be so vivid that it might generate an irresistible urge to enjoy the real thing. If so, you can scratch this particular trick from your repertoire. Most people, though, report that this exercise leaves them laughing and happy. Why not see how it works for you?

A final suggestion for avoiding feeling overwhelmingly deprived around food is to eat like a gourmet. Gourmets eat only the best. They wouldn't think of letting anything pass between their lips that was not really special. Gourmets also savor their food, getting maximum pleasure out of every marvelous

mouthful. They would never "inhale" their food, as I am sometimes wont to do. Eating a healthy diabetic diet doesn't mean
your palate has to go unpleased. When you please your palate,
those "I can't have anymore's" aren't nearly so painful.

June and Barbara: That's exactly the way we do it. We've
become such gastronomic fussbudgets that we do all of our
cooking and baking from scratch and even grow a lot of our
own vegetables. We absolutely never feel deprived on the "re-
stricted" diabetic diet.

But many diabetics who take the mourning band off their
sleeves for the food losses and changes still find it hard to
accept the loss of spontaneity in their lives. This is particularly true of young people on insulin. It's so disturbing to
them that sometimes they revolt and start doing what they
want to, when they want to, and let good diabetes control take
the hindmost. How can you help people adjust to this most
poignant of losses, the loss of spontaneity, and not just give up?

Dr. Rubin: Young diabetics complain about the loss of spontaneity almost as much as they do about food deprivations.
Several years ago I was treating Laura, a young diabetic
woman who worked in an office with lots of other young
single people. Since they were all footloose and fancy free,
they would often decide on the spur of the moment to go out
together after work. Typically, they would decide, as they
were leaving the building, to go someplace for dinner.

Laura was always prepared. She carried her insulin and
syringe in her purse. The only question was where to take her
shot. Much of the year this presented no problem—she did it
in her car before she went into the restaurant. But by late fall,
it was dark by the time she arrived at the restaurant. Have you
ever tried to draw up insulin with no illumination other than
one of those little 2-watt bulbs they put in car ceilings?

So she took her insulin into the restaurant restroom. When
she was in a hurry, she sometimes took her shot at the sink,
hoping no one would come in and think she was some sort of
junkie. Usually, though, she took all of her supplies into one of

the stalls. She'd place everything on the toilet paper roller. Public restroom toilet paper rollers are usually steady as a rock. They are engineered to save paper, and they turn very stiffly. Occasionally, though, Laura would come upon a loose roller, and her insulin and syringe would end up on the floor.

In spite of all the hassles involved, Laura always took her insulin before eating. Still, every time she joined her friends at the table after taking her shot, she thought, "What I'd give for just one day without that whole scene in the restroom."

This young woman dealt pretty constructively with the demands of her diabetes. Nobody's perfect; everyone rebels against the structure, restrictions, and lack of spontaneity from time to time. If your rebellions are occasional and short-lived, they are probably a healthy part of a grieving process that never ends.

But some people go further. They go beyond occasional rebellion to full-scale revolt—skipping shots, refusing to test for long periods, or completely trashing their diets. They get stuck in the denial or anger stages of grieving, unable to move on toward acceptance and healing.

June and Barbara: How do you help diabetics who are stuck in this state of revolt? We imagine that you see a number of them in your practice, since that's a problem that would logically lead a person to a therapist.

Dr. Rubin: Yes, I do see lots of them. When we start to work together, I begin by making one statement and asking one question. I tell them that I totally agree with their goal of living as free from diabetes as possible. Then I ask whether their approach actually accomplishes this goal. The answer is almost always no. That's not surprising, because revolting against diabetes actually gives the disease *more* control over your life. You feel sick and exhausted, so you can't do a lot of the things you want to do. You also spend more time in hospitals than you should. (Now, that's a really spontaneous experience.) And you're constantly haunted by guilt and fear, which does tend to put a damper on things.

June and Barbara: Since all this is true and obvious—so true and obvious that even people who are in the middle of revolt can see it themselves—why do they rebel?

Dr. Rubin: People don't revolt because it works; they revolt because they can't think of anything else to do. So it's our job to come up with something. The key is to trade in the decidedly mixed blessings of spontaneity for the more enduring benefits of flexibility. When you go for spontaneity you put your freedom before your health, and you end up with neither. When you go for flexibility, your freedom and your health become an inseparable package deal, and, if you play it smart, you end up with both.

June and Barbara: This sounds almost too good to be true. Could you give us a real-life example of how it works?

Dr. Rubin: OK. Lisa, a 17-year-old, came to me for treatment. Her hemoglobin A_{1c} scores had gone up several points over a period of six months, and she was missing quite a bit of school with minor ailments. Apparently, she and her friends went to the mall every evening and stuffed themselves with junk food. She didn't take her insulin with her on these search-and-consume missions because she didn't want the bother of finding a place to draw it up and give herself a shot. She convinced herself somehow that by the time she got home, "the damage was already done," so she didn't take a catch-up shot. She spent the night with sky-high blood sugars, making tracks from her bed to the bathroom and getting little sleep. In the morning she often felt so horrible that she couldn't drag herself to school.

Clearly, spontaneity wasn't working for this young lady. So we tried flexibility. She needed to maintain her mall munching (as far as Lisa was concerned, this was nonnegotiable) *and* she needed not to be tied down with insulin bottles, *and* she needed to get her diabetes back under control.

We brainstormed a bit before we hit on something Lisa was willing to try—carrying a predrawn syringe with three or four units of Regular insulin in her purse. This worked for her. Now the shot took no longer than going to the bathroom, and that she could live with. Don't ask me why the few seconds it took to draw up the insulin made so much difference; it just did. Or maybe carrying the bottle as well as the syringe was the straw that broke the camel's back. Who knows?

The point is that flexibility works where spontaneity doesn't. You just have to use your brains to find the solution that maximizes your freedom and your health. When you find it, your solution might be different from anyone else's, but that's what makes it so special.

June and Barbara: Does the arrival of complications such as loss of sight, being put on kidney dialysis, or having an amputation activate a new and different period of grief, and should this be handled differently?

Dr. Rubin: We've already talked about two kinds of diabetes-related grieving: grieving that follows being diagnosed diabetic, and grieving related to day-to-day losses, small and large. The onset of complications activates a third kind, which is unique in some ways.

Grieving over complications usually comes heavily mixed with guilt for all the transgressions, real and imagined, that led to the complications. In many ways, however, grieving over losses associated with complications is similar to other forms of diabetes-related grieving. People usually pass through the same stages of denial (shock), anger, depression, and bargaining before they ultimately reach acceptance.

June and Barbara: As always, we think it would help if you could give us a specific example from your own practice of this passage through the stages.

Dr. Rubin: I have many examples, but one woman who developed diabetic retinopathy gives a good picture of the process. Susan had received countless laser treatments over a period of years. Finally, it was clear that she needed more radical intervention to save her right eye, which had not responded well to laser treatments. Her doctors performed a vitrectomy, a procedure in which the vitreous humor (the transparent, gelatinous substance that fills the eyeball behind the crystalline lens) is replaced with saline solution. Susan had high hopes for the surgery, but in the weeks that followed, the doctors concluded that they had failed to save her eye.

At first, she was in a state of high denial, convinced that her vision was improving, that the surgery could be repeated with a better result, that other treatments must be available to save her eye. It took several months for Susan to accept the prognosis, and when she did, she got angry. She was mad at the surgeons for the poor result and for initially misleading her about the chances for success. She was mad at her endocrinologist for not keeping her under better control over the years so that she could have avoided this fate. She was mad at herself for not being a better patient.

Gradually, the anger began to ebb and depression took its place. She felt that her life was over. She was convinced that her appearance had suffered. She felt she wasn't good company because she was so preoccupied with her loss. She had trouble sticking with her part-time job and often spent the entire day alone in her room. She felt very low indeed. She bargained with her fate, replaying her experience and looking for some way, any way, to reverse what had happened.

Then slowly, over a period that lasted almost a year, Susan began to work through her loss, *feeling* it instead of fighting against it. She came out of her shell, began to spend time with other people, realized that she could actually think about other things, even enjoy herself. She was no longer completely defined by her lost eye. I knew the healing was well under way the day she said to me, "I used to think I would never get over losing my eye; now I think of it as a spare. I have to live my life and work really hard to keep my other eye."

Strangely enough, many people who have had diabetes for years grieve going on insulin as intensely as they would a complication. One man told me, "Once I went on insulin, my life stopped completely." Many people associate insulin with a loss of freedom or increased worries about reactions, so it's almost as if they were being diagnosed all over again.

June and Barbara: Certain jobs are forbidden to diabetics on insulin. When this realization sets in it can cause a tremendous sense of loss and grief. We know of one young man whose life-long dream was to become a marine. With the diagnosis of diabetes that dream was destroyed. Others face the very real chance of being dismissed from their jobs because of diabetes, and this would produce an even stronger sense of loss and grief, not to mention economic insecurity. What is a good adjustment process for such a crisis in personal and financial life?

Dr. Rubin: Sad to say, some people do lose their jobs when they are diagnosed diabetic. Others, like the young man you mentioned, have their dreams nipped in the bud. I feel horrible every time I talk to someone affected this way.

I know a policeman with nine years on the force, who was terrified that his diagnosis would mean losing his job. I know two newly diagnosed diabetics who had devoted years to getting licensed to fly. One was two weeks away from his goal, and the other had finally gotten his license six weeks before his diagnosis. They both faced the same bottom line: bye-bye license. The stories go on and on.

How do you cope with this kind of crisis? It's time to call in the Serenity Prayer. You must be familiar with it, but it's worth reconsidering here. It goes: "God grant me the serenity to accept the things I cannot change, the courage to change the things I can, and the wisdom to know the difference."

Let's start with the last phrase—the wisdom to know the difference between what you can change and what you can't. Is this loss you face negotiable? In some cases the answer is unequivocally no. You will not be allowed to fly a plane if you take insulin, unless accompanied by a licensed pilot at all times, and you will not be allowed to fly a plane commercially, period.

June and Barbara: The young would-be marine had trouble knowing the difference. Joining the service was totally non-negotiable, yet he spent years writing letters trying to make it otherwise. He wrote to us to see if we could help to get him accepted. Fortunately, not all cases are as nonnegotiable as this.

Dr. Rubin: Even in those cases that aren't so cut-and-dried, it often takes wisdom to uncover the facts. You might be able to keep your job as a policeman or fireman. These decisions depend on city and state laws and on departmental policies, so there's some variation in how things work. You may find that you can stay with the department in a different capacity from the one you had.

Once you have established the facts about what is and is not possible, you're ready to apply the rest of the Serenity Prayer. You must have the serenity to accept what you cannot change. I'm not saying you have to like it, or even accept it without doing some raging and crying first. Remember, we're talking about a process here. Acceptance and serenity is the goal. Anger and tears can be steps toward that goal, as long as you don't get stuck on those steps. What's natural and healthy as a stage in a process is neither natural nor healthy as a permanent end-point for that process.

Why should you strive for acceptance? What's wrong with staying angry and raging against your fate? It's a lousy, unfair fate, isn't it? Sure, it's unfair, but the die has been cast. If you're absolutely barred from some activity because of your diabetes, beating your head against the wall won't change that fact. And it will drain energy you need to complete the Serenity Prayer: having the courage to change the things you can change. Make no mistake about it, making the changes we're talking about takes lots of courage.

June and Barbara: Just where and how do you apply this courage?

Dr. Rubin: That depends on your personality and the specific circumstances of your situation. You might choose to fight for your job or the opportunity you are being denied. A man I know filed a suit to be reinstated in his job as a newspaper sports editor. Sometimes this kind of fight takes place on a broader front, lobbying legislators and the like. Efforts like this can be very frustrating, but they can sometimes be very rewarding.

As an alternative to fighting, you might look for a job or opportunity as close as possible to the one you've lost. This can be a positive choice if you can find reasonable alternatives to your first choice and you have the courage to accept a compromise.

Finally, you can apply your courage to working with the situation not as a disaster but as a challenge, or even an opportunity. What skills do you have that you might use in a new field? What other work would you really like to do? You might as well be creative and ambitious here. Life has handed you a lemon; maybe you can turn it into lemonade (sugar-free, of course).

June and Barbara: This is a little off the track of the grieving related to the diagnosis of diabetes and the loss of opportunities and activities that goes along with it, but it is, nonetheless, grieving that we have seen in action, and it can be very intense. This is the grieving that diabetics go through when they lose a long, close, successful relationship with a doctor through relocation, retirement, or death. Do you have some suggestions on how to handle this kind of loss?

Dr. Rubin: Funny you should ask that. My sister's endocrinologist, with whom she's had a wonderful relationship for the last 10 years, is moving out-of-state. In fact, many of the people I treat are patients of this same special physician, and they are all grieving. That makes perfect sense to me. They have lost something important—a wise and caring partner in their journey with diabetes. And saying farewell was not their choice, which makes the pain even more acute.

What advice do I give my sister and her fellow grievers? First, go ahead and feel sad. The depth of your grief reflects the importance this relationship holds for you. Surely it hurts to think of how much you are losing, but it's wonderful to think of how much you have had, and the two cannot be separated. Be thankful. You have been well cared for, and perhaps more important, you have learned to take good care of yourself.

Taking good care of yourself is exactly what you need to do now. Try to be positive and realistic. There are other good doctors out there, though none will be quite the same as the one you've lost. You will be the same person, though, and you are the one who found this wonderful doctor in the first place. It wasn't just luck. You used all your skills then, and you can do it again. So get to it. Use your present doctor and other diabetics you know as resources.

Once you've come up with two or three doctors who seem as if they might be good, meet with each of them for a kind of interview. Take your time in making a final decision; remember how important a choice this is. You have the standard of your current doctor relationship to give you some idea of what you're looking for. At the same time, give yourself a little time to adjust to the new physician before deciding he or she is not right for you. Good relationships, just like the one that's ending, tend to grow better with time.

➤ Help for Those Who Want to Help Diabetics

June and Barbara: What is the best way for friends and family to give support during the period or periods of grieving over the diagnosis and the continuous problems of living with diabetes?

Dr. Rubin: Since we know that grieving goes on and on, the need for skills to support our diabetic loved ones goes on and on, too. The foundation for all of them is the ability to be there for another person, which I mentioned before. As I said, being there means focusing on what the other person is feeling and what that person needs. Since none of us is a mind reader, the only way to know what's going on inside another person's heart and head is to listen to what the person says, ask questions, and listen to the answers. Does this sound too simple?

Well, I do tend to favor simple solutions, especially when they're the best. And this one is.

June and Barbara: Maybe an example would show us how this simple solution actually works in a typical, everyday diabetic grieving situation.

Dr. Rubin: Let's say your diabetic loved one is grieving over the loss of the freedom to eat a big piece of chocolate cake at the dinner party you just attended. He might say to you, "I felt so cheated when everyone else had dessert and I had to settle for a cup of coffee."

You have to watch yourself here. You may be tempted to respond with something like, "Well, you know you can't eat that stuff without sending your blood sugar through the roof." This response misses the point. Of course, he knows the cake would mess up his control; that's not what he was talking about. He was talking about feeling deprived.

June and Barbara: What should you say? What can make him feel better about not being able to eat the cake?

Dr. Rubin: How about, "I'll bet that was hard. I felt for you. That's why I passed on the cake myself" (assuming that you did). This lets him know that you heard him, felt for him, and did what you could to support him.

June and Barbara: But what if you ate the cake along with everyone else?

Dr. Rubin: You could ask a question like, "Would it have helped if I hadn't eaten the cake? I didn't even think of it, and I'm sorry I wasn't more sensitive to what you were feeling." You might add, "I know there's only so much I can do to make things easier for you, but I want to do everything I can."

You then might ask other questions. "Should we handle things differently in the future?" might be a good one. These questions and statements let your loved one know you are really there for him. You can't keep him from feeling bad, and he's not asking you to. You *are* giving one of the world's great gifts—real, heartfelt support.

Speaking of gifts, most people, diabetics included, love a spontaneous, thoughtful little something: a card, a flower, an unexpected phone call, a backrub, a movie together—the list is endless. Give a gift when your loved one is a little down, give a gift when your loved one is a little up, give a gift any time at all. Who knows, he or she might catch the gift-giving bug too, and you will probably be at the top of the list of giftees. This kind of support is especially nice. Even though it has nothing to do with diabetes per se, it's bound to help in that realm. When you love your diabetic, your diabetic feels good about himself or herself, and that helps the person take better care of diabetes.

June and Barbara: During the Gulf War we heard a radio interview with a grief therapist who was talking about how to help children who were disturbed by the war, particularly those who had a family member stationed in the Persian Gulf area. She mentioned that in the case of the death of a loved one, the real grief doesn't come for eight months to a year. Up to that time the bereaved is in too much of a state of shock to really feel the grief. If this holds true for diabetes grief, it would pose a difficult problem. After that length of time, most of a diabetic's friends expect him or her to be over the grieving and ready to go on with life. Yet this would be the time when the person needs help and support the most. How long can you logically expect it to take for a diabetic's grieving process to begin—and end? And how can you make sure you're giving the support that's needed, when it's needed?

Dr. Rubin: The point at which people are really hit by the fact that they have diabetes and start to grieve is probably a highly individual matter. Some people start the process right at diagnosis. Others are either in a state of shock or denial at first, and only begin to grieve after a few months have passed. For people who take insulin, the "honeymoon period" (a seeming cessation of diabetes right after insulin therapy begins) during which the diabetes is relatively easy to manage contributes to a delay in grieving. This is probably fortunate for most people (I think it was for Stefan), because it allows for a more gradual adjustment to life with diabetes. Other people tell me that they still haven't accepted the fact that they have diabetes, or begun to grieve, even though they were diagnosed 10 or 20 years ago, or longer.

The determining factors of the amount of time it takes to start and finish grieving seem to be the individual's personality style and the type and severity of early physical adjustment to diabetes.

One particularly good piece of research was done at the University of Pittsburgh Medical School. Children who had just been diagnosed were interviewed right at diagnosis and every six months for some years after. Their parents were also interviewed at the same times. The researchers found that in the months following the diagnosis, a substantial number of the children exhibited reactions that met the criteria for psychiatric disorder. Most of these reactions took the form of anxiety or depression. Apparently, these kids were grieving. By the end of the first year after diagnosis, almost all of these reactions had cleared up, indicating that the grieving process had resolved. Interestingly, many mothers went through a nearly identical grieving process, while fathers, almost without exception, did not. I'm not sure whether this should be attributed to male stoicism or to the fact that mothers might have been much more involved in day-to-day management of the diabetes.

At any rate, if you're really close to a diabetic you'll probably be able to identify the grief signals whenever they appear, early or late (even if they come and go)—and react accordingly, giving the support described above. Above all, you should try not to be irritated or impatient when grieving takes place or at how long it takes. At least, you should try not to show your irritation or impatience. An individual's grief has its own time and pace.

CHAPTER 6

FEAR
IF YOU HAVE FEARS,
PREPARE TO SHED THEM NOW

At an earlier period in her life, Barbara had an unusual way of dealing with fear and its fraternal twin, anxiety: she'd pass out as cold as a mackerel and as stiff as if the mackerel had rigor mortis. Because of the suddenness of the onset of the unconsciousness and her total rigidity from her clenched teeth to her clenched toes, Barbara was briefly misdiagnosed as being epileptic by one of the doctors in whose offices she performed this little fear-escaping technique. For that's what it was.

Whenever a doctor threatened her well-being with the merest suggestion that she might have a Dread Disease or could possibly need to have even minor surgery, Barbara would simply check herself out of the world. She would also check herself out on her own when she suffered something as inconsequential as feeling as if she might vomit or painfully banging her shin or elbow.

Once when we were going to speak at a diabetes conference at nearby California State University at Northridge, Barbara made the mistake of stubbornly taking an early morning jog despite the fact that she had the decided feeling she was coming down with the flu.

Later, at the conference, when we were sitting in the audience listening to the opening speaker, Barbara suddenly felt very sick. She whispered to June to stay there and take notes; she wasn't feeling too well and was going outside for a minute.

Barbara staggered up the aisle and out the door. The next thing June knew someone burst through the door shouting the legendary phrase, "Is there a doctor in the house?" June immediately knew what happened and had a vision (an accurate vision!) of Barbara doing her out cold and stiff number. But since there were about 25 doctors in the house and one hurried out to handle the crisis, June did as directed. She stayed put and continued to take notes.

The next thing Barbara knew someone was forcing her lips apart and trying to pour orange juice between them. Since this was a diabetes conference, the logical assumption was that she was a diabetic having an insulin reaction. The more Barbara protested that she was *not* a diabetic and did *not need* orange juice, the more the attending doctor figured she was a typical hypoglycemic diabetic fiercely fighting the very thing she needed to bring herself around. Finally, Barbara realized she had no choice. She choked down the glass of orange juice, thanked the doctor for his help, and sheepishly returned to the opening session.

Throughout the rest of the day, the major topic of conversation was "the poor diabetic woman who had passed out with a bad insulin reaction."

Effective as Barbara's passing out technique was for getting rid of fear, it was too short-lived to be of any real value. It could also be—as it was at the conference—extremely embarrassing and Barbara wanted to stop doing it. So, trained librarian that she was, she hit the books. She researched until she unearthed what it was that she was doing. It turned out that because she was so full of fear and anxiety, she unconsciously hyperventilated (breathed very rapidly). This blew off the carbon dioxide the body needs to activate the diaphragm, which controls breathing. The body defended itself by rendering her unconscious. Then her breathing would return to normal, the carbon dioxide balance would be restored, and she'd come to. (In her research Barbara discovered that the phenomenon was sometimes called the spoiled child syndrome, since children sometimes use this dramatically effective way to get their own way.)

The cure was easy. All she had to do was keep a paper bag handy in threatening places like doctors' offices. Whenever she felt herself starting to pass out, she would breathe into the bag. This restored the carbon dioxide balance without her passing out. Before long she found she could give up using the paper bag and just relax, control her breathing, and face up to her fears and deal with them like a big girl should.

We're telling you this not because we're suggesting hyperventilation as a temporary means of getting rid of your diabetes fears, but to show that knowledge and successful experience in applying that knowledge can help you handle fear.

Learning to handle fear can be a great asset. This was brought home to us by a story our accountant friend, Dorothy, told us about her early life. Dorothy was divorced and had put herself through college while supporting and caring for her son, who had been brain-damaged at birth. Before taking the CPA exam, she landed an entry-level job at a major accounting firm. She and the other new undocumented hirelings were given two weeks off to study for the exam. She studied in a cubicle at the office with one of the other female accountants. This woman was truly beautiful—almost movie star caliber. She came from a wealthy and influential family. Her father, who knew the higher-ups in the accounting firm, had got her the job without her having to go through the standard interview and screening procedures. Not that she needed his pull; on top of everything else, she was brilliant, an honors graduate of one of the best universities.

One day as they were studying, the woman raised her head and looked over at Dorothy. "You know," she said, "I really envy you."

Dorothy's jaw dropped. "There I was," she told us, "wearing no makeup, needing a haircut, clothes that were years old and not stylish to begin with, living in a dingy apartment, no money to speak of, and this woman who had everything and then some was saying she envied me."

"How could *you* possibly envy *me*?" Dorothy asked in amazement.

"You've had so many problems in your life and you've been able to handle them all," the woman said wistfully. "I know you can cope with anything that ever happens to you. I really envy that. I've always had everything so easy. Whatever I wanted just came to me with no effort. If I ever get hit with something really disastrous, I don't think I'll have the courage to handle it. I'm afraid I'll just go to pieces."

The moral is: if you gain the knowledge to help you conquer your many fears of diabetes, the courage that grows out of that will help you conquer other fears in your life.

One of our favorite aphorism writers, Mignon McLauglin, author of *The Neurotic's Notebook,* put it in her usual succinct way: "Courage can't see around corners, but goes around them anyway."

Dr. Rubin will now help you go around corners.

—June and Barbara

June and Barbara: Probably everyone who becomes diabetic has either a sudden or an on-and-off encounter with the fear of dying, because death now becomes not a remote possibility but a reality to be faced emotionally. This is a very sobering and maturing experience for most of us.

About a year after her diagnosis, June found herself thinking more and more about death and actually being somewhat terrified at the thought. "I had a recurring vision of myself as a helpless coward as I lay dying, unable to muster a shred of courage." Her reaction to this recurring vision was to start reading everything she could find on the subject. In the college library where we worked, we used to refer to her as "our death freak" and always referred students working on subjects like euthanasia or cryogenics (the freezing of bodies for later defrosting) to her. We knew a woman who was dying of cancer, and whereas most people felt uneasy with her and, if the truth be told, avoided her, June went out of her way to talk with the woman, letting her express her feelings and consoling her.

After about a year of her death apprenticeship, June was finally able to hold a picture in her mind of her own death as a calm and easy event. This attitude of tranquility has stayed with her ever since.

Have you found many diabetic patients with the same fears and intimations of mortality, and have they been able to work them out, as June was finally able to do, with positive results? Do you have suggestions for those who are still wrestling with this demon?

Dr. Rubin: People with diabetes spend a lot of time face to face with their mortality. How could it be otherwise? We all know we're going to die, but if you have diabetes, the frailties of the flesh are even more immediately apparent. Someone once called the ecstasy of sexual union "the little death," but this poetic phrase is probably better applied to the loss of consciousness that accompanies severe insulin reactions. Then there are the limitations and impositions of the regimen, which many people see as detracting from what it means to really live. Finally, and probably most powerfully, we face the specter of a life shortened and marked by physical disability.

Spending more time thinking about death than the average person is probably inevitable for the diabetic. In fact, this thinking can be positive, as it was for June. It can lead to a transcendent resolution; it can lead to an acceptance of death and a greater appreciation of life. Unfortunately, this outcome is relatively rare. Many people feel overwhelmed by these fears. They may even become obsessed with them. Why? Some people have very strong emotional constitutions. They're usually hardy and tend to use difficult experiences as opportunities to gain strength. Others are more vulnerable; they tend to be undone by the vicissitudes of life. Sometimes this vulnerability springs from painful experience. People who had older relatives with diabetes may be particularly susceptible to overwhelming fears of death associated with the disease. Memories or stories of blindness, amputated limbs, and death at an early age are bound to have an impact.

June and Barbara: We know many people with that kind of family background and it always seems to have an extremely negative influence on them and make it especially difficult for them to see their own situation as offering a totally different outcome.

Dr. Rubin: If they spend their time obsessing over fears of debilitation and an early death, the consequences are indeed very negative. First, their life is a whole lot less fun than it should be. Second, they risk creating a self-fulfilling prophecy. Intense worry has both direct and indirect effects on physical well-being. There's growing evidence that certain negative emotional states such as anxiety and depression are powerful risk factors for decreased longevity. And a strong belief that diabetes will kill you can contribute to a pattern of neglect that will almost certainly confirm your belief.

I'm reminded of Doug, a patient who was approaching his 35th birthday. His diabetes had been diagnosed when he was in his late teens, and he had never taken good care of himself. By some miracle he was still in decent health when he came to see me, confounded and dismayed by his inability to "do the right thing."

After a few sessions, we discovered that his father had died of diabetic complications at the age of 38 and that Doug had a powerfully held semiconscious belief that he, too, would die before he was 40. Once this belief was out in the open, we could talk about it. We discussed how it felt to be 10 years old and see your father die in raging denial of his disease—and how it felt now to have the same disease. We also talked about the ways in which Doug was different from his father, changes in the prognosis for people with diabetes, and the real choices he faced. These choices included living to see his own young sons grow up.

I have spent my entire adult life—30 years—associated with The Johns Hopkins University, and I have learned wisdom from its motto, *veritas vos liberabit.* "The truth will make you free" applies perfectly here. The truth of your own insides, emotional and physical, and the truth of what it really means to have diabetes now, not 20 or 30 years ago, will make you free to choose your own life with this disease.

June and Barbara: Is this fear of early death and complications always a totally negative force? We've seen it work to shape people up and get them to improve their diabetes control when nothing else could.

Dr. Rubin: Fear of complications can be a positive force if it motivates you to take good care of yourself. Using the prospect of complications to your advantage requires a delicate intellectual and emotional balancing act. On the one hand, you must recognize and accept the reality of complications; they can strike diabetics, especially those who have lived with the disease for many years. On the other hand, you must recognize and accept the fact that complications are not inevitable. Every day evidence mounts that you can greatly improve your odds of delaying complications or avoiding them altogether if you maintain good control. And every day new technology emerges that makes it easier to achieve good control.

This kind of balancing act isn't easy, so many people tend to deal with the prospect of complications in a way that makes it a negative force. Instead of balancing the reality of complications and the possibility of avoiding them, these people slide to one extreme or the other. They either try to deny the reality of complications, acting as if they're immune, or they're fatalistic, acting as if there's no escape. Coming from opposite directions, each of these approaches leads to the same destructive behavior. If you're immune to complications, you don't have to do anything to avoid them; if you're bound to get complications no matter what you do, it doesn't matter what you do. As destructive as these attitudes are, it's not hard to understand why they develop. Complications are scary, so an attitude of denial or "ignorance is bliss" seems to offer some comfort. But as one of my patients said, "I've spent the six years since my diagnosis living in ignorance, but for me ignorance is not bliss, because I can't escape the fear of losing my eyesight." This underlines a point I made earlier: denial doesn't work well, because it is rarely complete. There's almost always a crack, and even a little crack is enough to let the fear in.

What is really hard to do is create the kind of balanced view of complications that turns the fear of them into a positive force. In my experience, this kind of view usually comes later, when complications are no longer a dreaded specter but a painful reality. At this point, many people are finally "scared straight."

June and Barbara: Surely there's some way to help people deal constructively with these fears without waiting until they actually have complications.

Dr. Rubin: What you can do is keep reminding yourself of the facts I mentioned above:

1. Your power to control your blood sugar is growing every day with new technologies.

2. The better care you take of yourself now, the more likely you are to be in good shape when the cure finally comes.

3. Remind yourself that the fate of older diabetics need not be your fate.

Beyond this, you need to think of the thoughts or images that can motivate you. For some people, one particular complication scares them more than all others. Perhaps this could be a motivator. One man told me, "Every day I worry that I'll have to go on the dialysis machine for my kidneys." My son listened without reacting as I told him about all the complications that can strike a diabetic, until I mentioned impotence. He stopped me there with the comment, "If you ever want to scare me straight, that's the one to mention." As always, the proof of the pudding is in the eating. So you might try this trick of bringing to mind your most dreaded complication, perhaps in combination with the thought that you can avoid this fate, and see if it does motivate you.

June and Barbara: As a former librarian and avid reader who considers her eyes among her most precious commodities, June has always been highly motivated by her desire to prevent blindness.

Dr. Rubin: Most people, however, are more motivated by positive images. You can use the prospect of complications to your advantage by picturing yourself free of them. Imagine yourself as a hale and hardy 85-year-old hiking, swimming, and running rings around people 20 years younger. Then tell yourself that you can be that way *if* you take good care of yourself.

No one can guarantee you'll be free of complications if you maintain good control or that you'll definitely get them if you don't. But it's like driving a car with an air bag compared with a car that doesn't even have a seatbelt. The odds of surviving a crash are very different. What it's all about is accepting the fact that you could get complications but that you can influence the likelihood that you won't get them.

June and Barbara: Among Type II diabetics the greatest and most common fear—maybe we should say terror—is the threat of having to take insulin. In many cases it's a pathological dread. How do you counsel these people and help them escape this needless agony?

Dr. Rubin: You're right, this is a big fear. One man said to me, "I know my diabetes is out of control, but I just hate the prospect of taking needles. I'd rather take cyanide." Fairly dramatic, no? As you point out, this is not an isolated comment. Many diabetics respond to the prospect of insulin as if they had gotten diabetes all over again, only worse this time.

What in the world is going on here? Is it fear of needles? This is probably part of it, and the part most people have the easiest time expressing, but I don't think it's the whole story for anyone. Here are the other factors involved.

Guilt: For some people guilt is an element in this intense reaction. Many people feel they are faced with insulin because they failed to manage their diabetes with diet and oral medication. Starting on insulin is a confirmation of this failure.

Diabetes getting worse: Some people think that having to take insulin means their diabetes is getting worse, and that's an unwelcome and scary thought.

Harder regimen: There's extra work involved in a regimen that includes insulin. Planning and scheduling are more critical to success and there are more factors to juggle.

Insulin reactions: Taking insulin greatly increases the likelihood of insulin reactions, and these episodes are anticipated with dread.

For a given person the fear of going on insulin can be the result of any or all of these factors. When people come to me for counseling because they're panicked, I start by helping them identify which of the factors apply to them. (Sometimes they come up with others unique to them.) Then we work to deal with the specific thoughts and feelings that trigger their fears of insulin.

June and Barbara: Can you analyze them for us one by one?

Dr. Rubin: They include:
Fear of needles. The morbid fear of needles is called acuphobia. We might start by identifying the place where

it would feel least horrible to give the shot. Most people can tell you where that is, even before they've ever had an injection. Then, I tell the person to administer all shots there until the process is a little less scary. I might also give myself a shot with sterile water in front of them. I might relate different things people do to make shots less frightening, such as injecting very slowly or very fast, or having someone else do it at first. Basically, I offer a menu of things that might help, and my patient decides what to try. In my experience, this kind of desensitization process usually doesn't take long.

Guilt: For those who feel guilty about having taken such poor care of themselves that they must take insulin, I start by helping the patient acknowledge these feelings. The fact is, sometimes going on insulin *is* the result of not doing everything you could to work with diet, exercise, and oral medication. If that's the case, maybe the prospect or reality of taking insulin will help you locate the motivation that has been missing. Maybe that could lead to avoiding insulin or to going off it after a short while.

Diabetes getting worse: Going on insulin doesn't mean that the diabetes is getting worse. I make that clear to people who express this concern. Diabetes is diabetes. Getting worse can only be measured in terms of blood-sugar control or complications, and, in that sense, going on insulin can actually lead to diabetes getting *better.*

Harder regime: Life is more complicated when you take insulin than when you manage your diabetes by diet or oral medication. I won't argue that for a moment. I just listen to the disappointment, frustration, and fear people express when they talk about the additional demands and limitations. Letting them vent these feelings tends to relieve them to a certain degree.

Insulin reactions: These are a major source of legitimate concern. Talking about how to prevent or handle them is the best we can do on this one.

People have a right and a need to be upset and scared about their new regime. What they also need to keep in mind, which I'm here to help them do, is that there are benefits as well as costs associated with taking insulin. I'll talk about the long-term benefits, to be sure, but the more immediate benefits are often more salient. With patients who are not yet on insulin, I'll ask them how they're feeling. The answer is usually, "Terrible," once we get down to reality. Then I'll make the point that this terribleness is probably closely related to high blood sugars and that it will be relieved by the use of insulin for improved glucose control. If they've already started on insulin, I simply help them focus on how much better they feel physically than they did before they made the switch.

June and Barbara: For someone who has fear and loathing for the needle, this may seem like a ridiculous suggestion, but it worked for June. She started taking more shots a day. She did this to improve her diabetes control and give herself more flexibility in her lifestyle, but a fringe benefit was that she didn't dread taking her shots as much as she had in the past. She said it seemed as if she didn't have as much time between shots to fret about having to take the next one. It did, indeed, become more routine, although it has never become like brushing your teeth, the way some health professionals claim it will once you get used to it. (She now takes five shots a day, but two of them are with a needleless jet injector.)

Dr. Rubin: That makes a lot of sense to me on two counts. First, taking shots more often can make the process seem more routine. People seem to have an easier time accommodating themselves to things they have to do often. Maybe part of the explanation is the time interval between shots. Much of the fear may be in the anticipation. I certainly felt this was true for my son during a period when he would sit with the needle poised over his arm for what seemed like hours. Finally, he would press it ever so slowly into his flesh. I was reminded of old science fiction movies with slow-motion shots of spaceships docking. The whole process was agonizing for him, and I was convinced, though he was not, that his fear and pain were directly proportional to the amount of time he took.

Another factor might account for some of the fear reduction associated with more frequent shots. More frequent shots may mean more stable blood sugars, fewer reactions, and less fear of the whole insulin administration process. This possibility relates to June's initial motivation for taking shots more often—improved diabetes control and a more flexible lifestyle.

By the way, I'm not surprised that June has never gotten to the point where her shots are as easy as brushing her teeth. Given the choice between these two activities, anyone who would pick the shots is probably in need of my professional services.

June and Barbara: Several times we've encountered people who have had diabetes for a number of years and have been giving themselves insulin injections with no fear or difficulty, and yet when they start taking their blood sugar, they're terrified and can hardly bring themselves to stick their fingers. Is this because sticking your finger and seeing the blood involves a different kind of fear? Are you more likely to feel you're wounding yourself? Is the sight of blood, especially your own, often more frightening than sticking yourself with an insulin needle? Have you found more men frightened of insulin injections and more women frightened of the finger stick, or vice versa, or is it about the same?

Dr. Rubin: I'll answer the last question first. I've never noticed any differences between men and women in these fears. Your question is intriguing, though. I'll start paying more attention.

I *have* met many diabetics who say they hate finger sticks much more than they do insulin injections. I think there may be several reasons for this:

1. The sight of blood is very disturbing for some people.

2. Many people say that finger sticks hurt more. They say that the stick itself is more painful and that there's more soreness afterwards, especially if you do the stick on the pad of your finger, which comes into contact with practically everything when you're using your hands.

3. If you don't get a large enough drop of blood when you stick yourself, you either have to do it again or sit there milking your finger for what seems like an eternity. I recently read a great hint in a medical journal for getting a good drop of blood. Just before you stick yourself, wrap a rubber band (not too tightly) around the first joint of your finger. When you're done with the test, take the rubber band off right way. I mentioned this technique to a teenager who was having problems with his drops, and he reported that it worked almost too well. When he stuck his finger he got a little geyser of blood that made him thankful he was wearing glasses. But the technique made him test more often than he had been.

4. When some people say they fear finger sticking, what they really mean is that they fear seeing high blood-sugar readings. This is my hypothesis and soon I hope to have a way of testing it.

A new technology on the way will use infrared light to measure blood sugar. These meters will read right through the skin, with no finger stick required. Plus, they give an instantaneous reading. I used one of these prototype meters recently, and sure enough, I didn't feel a thing. So if what you really hate is the result of your test, you'll soon have to come clean and face the truth.

The history of this technology is interesting, too. It originated from agricultural research. Growers of fruit wanted to know how ripe their crops were (measured by sugar levels) without cutting open the fruit. Scientists developed a technique to do just that. One of these researchers was in England a few years ago, and he was interviewed about his work on a radio talk show. After the show a woman called the scientist, saying she had a diabetic daughter and asking whether this same technique could be used to measure blood-sugar levels. The rest, as they say, is history.

June and Barbara: There is one particularly torturing fear that virtually all insulin-taking diabetics suffer from to a greater or lesser degree: the fear of insulin reactions (also called hypoglycemia or insulin shock). Whether you're in tight control or totally out of control, insulin reactions are an ongoing hazard and constant threat.

What has amazed us most is that we've met many newly diagnosed diabetics who were carefully instructed in how to give themselves injections of insulin, but they received no warning or information on how to handle insulin reactions. A few people have told us about learning what an insulin reaction is by having one. Imagine the fear that such a mysterious and unexpected experience can engender. As we all know, a fear once implanted in the mind is not easily dismissed.

To us the fear of insulin reactions is a normal and healthy fear, one that leads most insulin-takers to exercise the necessary precautions to avoid dangerous accidents and damaging bouts of unconsciousness. But when a truly terrifying incident takes place without warning and with no logical explanation, the fear that takes hold afterward may refuse to go away. A nocturnal episode of unconsciousness can make you afraid to go to sleep at night. Parents often can't sleep because they're worried that their diabetic child will go into a serious reaction without their knowing it. Adults who have had automobile accidents because of low blood sugar have been afraid to drive a car again.

Large numbers of diabetics suffer routinely from what is now being called hypoglycemic unawareness. This means they get no signals at all that they're below, say, 50 mg/dl (2.7 mmol/L).

I'm sure you're even more aware than we are of the mental distress that insulin reactions cause. How can people cope with this fear and learn to keep it in perspective?

Dr. Rubin: As you point out, fear of insulin reactions is a normal and healthy fear. Reactions are the most unpleasant and potentially serious short-term complication of diabetes. The most common symptoms of a reaction include: trembling, pounding heart, shaking hands, difficulty concentrating, confusion, and poor physical coordination. Reactions are also embarrassing. They can even be dangerous, if they lead to unconsciousness. For all these reasons, you must take sensible precautions to minimize them. Unfortunately, some people are so terrified of low blood sugars that they avoid them at all costs, even the cost of running dangerously high all the time.

Running chronically high blood sugars is tempting if you're really afraid of reactions. After all, day-to-day you probably won't notice any serious side-effects. Maybe you'll have to urinate several times a night, feel tired a lot, and maybe your vision will be blurry from time to time, but what's that compared to feeling free from worry about falling down in public or running your car into a tree in the throes of a reaction? From this perspective, running high makes quite a bit of sense.

Unfortunately, this isn't the only perspective that applies. Chronically high blood sugars have their consequences, too. The most serious ones are not immediate but long-term. I guess it's only human to respond more powerfully to bad things in the present than to the prospect of bad things in the future, especially when the former takes so much less effort than the latter. But in this case what's natural and easier is not what's good for you.

June and Barbara: Agreed! We all understand this great dilemma and that it's a universally felt fear. So what do we do?

Dr. Rubin: You're caught between a rock and a hard place. There's no easy solution to this dilemma. I'm not here to tell you otherwise. I can offer three suggestions I've picked up from people who seem to be having some success with this balancing act.

1. **Always be prepared for reactions.** This may sound ridiculously obvious, but many people just don't do it. *Always* carry an antidote. Have glucose tablets (Dextrosols, Dextrotabs, or B-Ds) in your pocket or purse, in your car, with your sports gear, and by your bed at all times. If you can treat your reactions instantly you'll fear them less.

You also need to be prepared for those times when a reaction sneaks up on you or is so intense that you can't treat it yourself. Carry some form of diabetes identification such as a bracelet or wallet card. Be sure that people you spend lots of time with know what to do for you. Be sure you have glucagon (a prescription drug; the hormone that raises blood sugar) available and that your family has been taught when, how, and where to inject it.

All these precautions can help contain reactions and protect you from experiences that may make you phobic and lead you to the dangerous conclusion that chronically high blood sugars are your only safe choice.

2. **Know yourself.** This isn't as obvious as it might seem. Your fears are specific to you and so are your solutions. Have you ever had a really traumatic low-blood-sugar experience? Do you tend to have reactions without warning (hypoglycemic unawareness)? If you answered yes to either of these questions, you need to work harder than most people to avoid reactions.

One patient of mine often had severe reactions without warning. Her solution was to test her blood sugar every time she was about to get into her car and before certain crucial work-related activities. Was all this testing bothersome? Sure it was, but as she put it, "It certainly beats either ending up in some terrible car accident that I caused or finding myself on dialysis in 10 years."

A colleague of mine at the University of Virginia studies how people deal with their fears of hypoglycemia. Based on this work, he's set up an experimental program to train people in low-blood-sugar awareness in the hopes that increased awareness will lead to improved self-care and physical and emotional well-being. He's hoping to help even those people whose awareness of hypoglycemia is very low.

3. **Let the situation guide you.** In circumstances where a reaction would be particularly unwelcome, such as during a job interview or an exam, it might make sense to run a bit high. This gets tricky, of course, since these same situations might trigger stress-hormone-induced high blood sugar anyway, and being *really* high creates its own problems. This is another time when you have to know your own body and how it tends to operate.

All in all, the best guidance I've heard boils down to being prepared, knowing your own body, and being flexible. I guess that's good advice for living in general as well as for living with diabetes.

June and Barbara: A young man we know says that his biggest problem with diabetes is resisting the temptation to eat everything in sight when he's in the throes of a reaction. Once he's done this, his blood sugar skyrockets and he spends most of the rest of the day feeling horrible and trying to get back under control. He knows he's doing the wrong thing, but he just can't seem to stop. What's going on and what can he do about it?

Dr. Rubin: This problem, which is not at all uncommon, has a variety of causes. First, reactions are often extremely uncomfortable, so there's a natural human tendency to keep eating until you feel better. Since it takes a while for whatever you eat to take hold, it's easy to end up overdoing the treatment. Even after your blood sugar has been brought up to normal, your symptoms, especially hunger, are likely to persist for at least fifteen minutes to half an hour.

Another reason for overtreating is the fact that hypoglycemia often leads to a confused mental state. In this state, everything you know about what you should do goes right out the window, and your mind operates at its most primitive level, screaming, "Eat! Eat!"

Overtreating reactions can also be part of a learned pattern. One of my patients who has strong tendencies in this direction says that she began overtreating when she was a teenager right after she was diagnosed. Helen's rule was "*Never have a reaction.*" She was determined that her friends would never look at her funny and that she would never find herself unable to run laps and risk being cut from the sports teams she loved so much. Her solution was to stuff herself in any situation where a reaction was even a slight possibility. She told me that for years her attitude was "I've got these guys [the doctors] fooled." She completely avoided reactions. She didn't even have to worry about having a nighttime snack. No wonder, her blood sugars were probably over 200 all the time.

Helen became a nurse, working on a service that demanded constant alertness. This only reinforced her pattern. On those rare occasions when her blood sugar got low, she felt she couldn't follow her doctor's advice to take a little juice and a few crackers and sit for 15 minutes. In 15 minutes one of her patients might die! So she would consume many times the calories needed to correct her blood sugar and fly back into action.

Today Helen is suffering from complications, probably partly as a result of her tendency to run high to avoid reactions. She still struggles with her temptation to eat out of control when she's low, and we're working together to help her solve this problem. One approach she's trying is to prepare a care package containing just enough food to effectively treat most reactions. This has helped. Instead of going to the refrigerator on a search-and-consume mission, she now picks up her care package, sits down and eats it, and waits for 15 minutes to see how she's doing. (She's no longer working the demanding nursing job.)

Another approach Helen has tried is to use one of the pre-packaged antireaction agents (Insta-Glucose, Monoject Reaction Gel, Glutose) instead of food. She dislikes the taste of these products, so she is much less likely to overtreat when she uses them. Finally, we have worked out a little mantra for her to repeat as she waits the 15 minutes to see how her blood sugar is doing. It goes like this: "Relax, you'll be fine. You can wait a little. You'll be fine." The key here is to keep the message to yourself reassuring and simple. If it has a critical edge or gets too complicated, it won't work, given your vulnerable state.

June and Barbara: Here's a fear that one of our readers asked us about after reading *The Diabetic Woman:* "I thought you might be interested in a small problem of mine that comes from growing up with diabetes. I find I am very reluctant to increase my insulin dosage, even if I need to. In part this is due to the thought that more medication means I'm not as healthy. Part of the problem, I believe, stems from my adolescence. During my early and middle teen years I was taking a lot of insulin. I believe my all-time high was close to 80 units per day. I very often encountered shocked expressions from health professionals when they said, 'My, you're taking a lot of insulin, aren't you?' I felt helpless and abnormal and to this day have to consciously force myself to increase my dosage when necessary." June had to confess that she, too, even without the help of health professionals, automatically finds herself interpreting needed dose increases in the same way. Intellectually she knows this is nonsense, because all that matters is how good control is as measured by hemoglobin A_{1c}, and not how large the dose is. But still, like this reader, she can't seem to dismiss her feelings easily. She's reluctant to increase her dosage when necessary and sometimes delays doing it.

On the other hand, when it looks as if her insulin needs are going down, she makes the reduction immediately. Can you tell us how diabetics who think this way can assuage their feelings about increases and stop these negative perceptions?

Dr. Rubin: The number of people I meet who measure "how bad" their diabetes is by the amount of insulin or the number of shots they take is legion. But when I ask someone who holds this belief to explain it to me, we usually end up where June does, recognizing that the diabetes of someone who maintains good control with 40 units a day in five shots is generally no worse than the diabetes of someone who maintains the same level of control with 20 units in two shots. The gauge of how bad or good your diabetes is is your physical and emotional well-being, not the type, timing, and amount of insulin you take. In fact, of course, people who take more shots a day may be maintaining better control than those who take fewer, and those who take enough insulin to maintain good control are certainly healthier than those who don't take enough.

I should point out one qualification here. While it's wise to take enough insulin to maintain good control, it's also wise to take the least amount of insulin you can to achieve that control and to rely as much as possible on exercise and healthy eating to hold down your insulin needs. This makes sense in terms of a balanced approach to self-care. There's some evidence, too, that high levels of circulating insulin in the blood may contribute to increased risk of cardiovascular disease. Not only that, but insulin is a potent fat-building hormone, so someone with a weight problem wouldn't want to shoot up a lot of insulin to cover extra food. The bottom line is that the amount of insulin you take does not reflect how bad your diabetes is, but taking more insulin shouldn't be your only approach to good control.

June and Barbara: How do you get rid of an irrational belief that the goodness or badness of diabetes can be measured by the regimen used to treat it?

Dr. Rubin: You just have to listen to your body, hear without fear or preconceptions what it tells you it needs, and love it by giving it what it needs. If you need to go on insulin, your body will tell you. Your blood sugars will be high, despite your best efforts to control them with diet, exercise, and oral medication, and you'll feel the effects of those high blood sugars. Those effects are uncomfortable in themselves, and they are your body's attempt to let you know it's hurting, that it can't keep taking care of you unless you find some better way to take care of it. Much the same thing will happen if you're already taking insulin and you need more. Increasing the number of shots you take may be a different matter. It might be directed toward smoothing out your blood sugars by redistributing the insulin you take, rather than increasing the total amount. Changing your regimen doesn't mean that your diabetes is worse, but not changing your regimen may well mean that your diabetes *will* get worse.

June and Barbara: Among adolescents, the fear of being different is a major cause of neglecting diabetes self-care. Is there any approach that can be taken to help them avoid behaviors that are in the long run extremely self-destructive?

Dr. Rubin: I'd say this fear of being different is common in people of all ages, though perhaps it is most common during adolescence, when being different is particularly painful. The approach I suggest is to figure out ways to manage your diabetes that create as few differences as possible. Let's look at some of the main sources of feeling different and see how this might work. The things I hear mentioned most often are:

> ➤ Inability to participate in social activities, sports, and other activities as spontaneously and easily as everyone else.
> ➤ Awkwardness in situations involving food.
> ➤ Discomfort associated with testing and taking shots.
> ➤ Limitations imposed by low and high blood sugars.

To minimize feeling different in any given situation, imagine a balance. On one side are your diabetes self-care needs and on the other your social fitting-in needs. If you put everything on either side of the balance—ignoring your diabetes or your social needs—your life will be pulled unmanageably off-center. If you insist on always eating exactly the right thing at exactly the right time, for instance, you're almost sure to feel different from other people. (Maybe that's okay with you, and maybe it isn't.) Ironically, going to the other extreme can also lead to feeling different. If you ignore your diabetes—not taking your insulin or eating when you should, for example—you may well end up feeling really sick from high blood sugar or an insulin reaction. Having your blood sugars out of whack is guaranteed to make you acutely aware you have diabetes and other people don't. To avoid these imbalances, you need to respect both sets of needs. Otherwise, one or the other of them is going to get you.

June and Barbara: What does it mean to have a recurring nightmare about forgetting or losing your insulin?

Dr. Rubin: I've never heard this one before. Was this one of your dreams, June? I'd like to know before I put my foot in my mouth with some exotic interpretation based on repressed anal-retentive tendencies.

June and Barbara: Yes, it was, or we should say is. June has this dream about as frequently as she used to have one about forgetting to show up for a final exam in college.

Dr. Rubin: I was just joking. Actually, attaching meanings to dreams can be a pretty tricky business. This one is relatively straightforward, however. If we take it fairly literally, the dream tells us that the dreamer has some fears about her diabetes, particularly about juggling all the things that need to be balanced to maintain good control. These things create a certain edge of anxiety, even when they're all managed well. I wouldn't be surprised to hear that June wasn't particularly aware of this anxiety in her waking state. That's what dreams are for: they tell us about those feelings we tend to pay less attention to while we're awake. Since insulin is one of the most crucial elements of the regimen, it makes sense that insulin would be the symbol brought to mind in the dream, even if it was never actually lost or forgotten in waking reality. The fear of losing or forgetting insulin represents the fear that the whole regimen might become unmanageable. Again, let me emphasize that this is not a full representation of reality. Dreams don't reveal a deeper level of truth. They simply reveal an aspect of truth that wasn't fully acknowledged by the waking mind.

At a deeper level, this is a more general dream about control, and the fear of losing it. Many people have dreams about forgetting or losing important things—appointments, plane flights, keys, people's names, where they parked their car. The list is almost endless. My own most popular theme for this type of dream is forgetting when I'm supposed to be at an airport. In the dream I spend forever locating my tickets, only to realize that my flight leaves in 15 minutes and I'm in my hotel with nothing packed and various family members wondering why I'm not at the gate. At this more general level, the insulin is just another personally relevant important thing, and the fear of losing or forgetting it reflects a basic human fear that things may come undone.

June and Barbara: People sometimes have a great fear that they'll lose their jobs if their employer finds out they're diabetic. Is this realistic and if so, what is the best way for diabetics to overcome this particular kind of fear?

Dr. Rubin: This is a tough question to answer. Start by sorting out exactly what you're afraid of, because the best course of action depends on the specific fear you're dealing with. Here are some job situations about which I've heard diabetics express fears.

1. Jobs that are forbidden to diabetics in general or to insulin-treated diabetics in particular.

As we mentioned in the grief chapter, some jobs are clearly not available to diabetics, at least not to those who take insulin. The military, interstate trucking and busing, airline piloting, and a few others are forbidden by federal law to insulin-treated diabetics. Whatever the pros and cons of these restrictions, no diabetic should try to hide his or her condition in these cases. You won't be able to get away with it, and it's too dangerous to try. You just have to grieve the loss of opportunity, and it can be a real and very painful loss to you.

2. Jobs where you would be at risk simply by revealing you have diabetes.

In these cases, first think about what it will cost you to hide your diabetes. If you don't take insulin, and don't have reactions, the cost might be fairly low. If you do take insulin the cost might be much greater. Will you have to run high all the time to avoid reactions and discovery? Will you feel uncomfortable having to keep secret an essential fact about yourself? If you tell someone at work, will that person honor your confidence or will word get back to your boss? What will happen if your boss finds out about your diabetes in this way? Will you ever be required to take a physical that will reveal diabetes? Will you ever make insurance claims for diabetes-related services that might come to the attention of your employer?

I am biased toward being open about having diabetes. I'd want to educate my employer about diabetes. But I can safely take this radical position. Maybe you really want this job, maybe you know what the employer's attitude will be. If you believe you can keep your secret without paying too heavy a price, give it a try. Your sense of the benefits and costs of your decision might change as time passes.

3. Jobs where there is a prejudice against people with diabetes or even simply an extreme insensitivity to their needs.

Will you have problems about taking breaks for snacks, doing blood tests, treating reactions, doctors' appointments, and the like? You have to weigh the risks not only of revealing your diabetes but of asking for the flexibility in your schedule to deal effectively with your self-care. In most cases, the risk of asking for time for your needs is the greater risk. Most bosses are concerned with the so-called bottom line. They worry about your productivity and their profits.

Now we come to the feeling you may have that you're a victim of outright discrimination. The 1990 Americans with Disabilities Act pretty much outlaws discrimination against diabetics in the workplace. Employers with more than 15 employees aren't even allowed to ask if you have diabetes when you apply for a job, and they're required to make reasonable accommodation for your special needs. If you meet with discrimination, contact your state American Diabetes Association affiliate for help.

As a final antidote to fear in the workplace, I want to reassure you that sick days are there to be used when you're sick. The fact that you use most of your days for diabetes-related problems is no one's business but yours. A woman who worked as a teacher worried every time she took a sick day on account of diabetes. She was "paranoid they are going to lay me off." Of course, it's up to you not to let your diabetes have a substantial impact on your job performance. Try to figure out what's going on. If the basic problem is how you're caring for your diabetes, if you get that straightened out, you'll have addressed your job-related fears as well.

A related job issue is health insurance. One woman I treated was considering a job change, but her current employer provided excellent health-care coverage. If she changed jobs, she had no idea what kind of coverage she would have. As she put it, "What happens if I get less coverage and my medical problems get worse?" This is a critical question and one she must ponder carefully. That's a fact of life with diabetes. All she can do is assess it carefully and feel angry because her diabetes makes this an important factor, and then make her choice accordingly.

June and Barbara: A stock trader friend of ours told us that a year before he was diagnosed diabetic he had terrible panic attacks that would come on him suddenly and for no apparent reason. He was exercising regularly and eating a fairly healthy diet. He was under some stress at work, but nothing unusual. His doctor sent him to a psychiatrist. That didn't help. Once he was diagnosed diabetic and started taking insulin, the attacks went away, never to return.

According to the book *The Good News About Panic, Anxiety, and Phobias* by Dr. Mark S. Gold, panic attacks can be caused by fluctuations in blood sugar, and this might explain our friend's experience. Have any patients come to you because of panic attacks either prior to diagnosis or when their blood sugars were out of control? Did stabilizing blood sugar eliminate the attacks, or did these patients need counseling, too?

Dr. Rubin: In my experience panic attacks related to undiagnosed diabetes are quite rare. Undiagnosed diabetes signifies high blood sugar, and most of the diabetics I treat feel less anxious with blood sugars a little on the high side. There seem to be a couple of reasons for this tendency. First, some people actually like the feeling of being a bit slowed down by high blood sugar. They say it kind of mellows them out. One young college student I was treating told me she always let herself run higher than usual just before exams. She knew she wasn't quite as sharp for studying, but she felt much more relaxed, as if she'd taken a Valium, and the tradeoff worked for her.

Much more commonly people let themselves run on the high side because, for them, panic attacks related to blood-sugar levels are triggered by lows rather than highs. This makes good sense, because panic attacks are always triggered by physical symptoms. The mind sees the symptoms as threatening and creates the feeling of panic. It's the meaning the mind gives the symptoms that causes the terror. When blood sugar gets too low, first you have the physical sensation stage—headache, sweating, shakiness, confusion, pounding heart, difficulty concentrating. These feeling are uncomfortable, sometimes extremely so. Notice, too, that some of these sensations are identical to those we feel when we're anxious and under major stress. That's because these sensations are triggered by the release of stress hormones, the body's natural attempt to rally from a low blood sugar.

Then comes the mental stage, the feeling of panic and losing control. The activation of the stress hormones opens the door to feeling panicky, and so does awareness that having a low-blood-sugar reaction can be a serious or even life-threatening situation. The mind takes that idea and runs with it.

Treatment for these panic attacks is generally unnecessary. Once people realize what their physical sensations really mean and don't mean, they almost always stop misinterpreting their symptoms in ways that lead to panic. Occasionally people will continue to attach some dread meaning to their symptoms or to the fact they have diabetes. In such cases I help them discover what these meanings are and how to take away their power. Sometimes this meaning is fairly easily discovered and disarmed. For some these fears are based on outdated ideas about the inevitable fate of a person with diabetes. On rare occasions the situation is harder to resolve, though these are almost always cases in which diabetes is only one of a mountain of serious problems the person is facing.

➤ Help for Those Who Want to Help Diabetics

June and Barbara: Just as they say you can't love someone else unless you learn to love yourself, you can't help assuage another person's fears until you come to terms with your own. As Dr. Rubin pointed out in this chapter, some of the most disturbing and detrimental things a diabetic's loved ones do stem from their own fears.

The basic way to overcome your own fears is the same way diabetics overcome their fears: through learning as much as you can about diabetes. Not only will this knowledge help set you free from your fears, it will make what you say have more clout with your diabetic loved one. For example, just saying something like, "Don't worry, everything will be fine, you won't have any of those terrible complications" or "Don't worry, you can have a baby and it will be perfectly normal" will have very little fear-alleviating impact. On the other hand, if you can reinforce your positive prognostications with back-up documentation based on your reading and on the information you've gained in diabetes classes and meetings of diabetes associations, what you say will have reassuring credibility.

Dr. Rubin, besides learning as much as possible about diabetes, have you found other ways to help a diabetic's loved ones overcome their own fears?

Dr. Rubin: I think education is the foundation for dealing with diabetes-related fears, but knowledge alone is not enough. Once you feel that you know what you need to know about diabetes and its treatment, you can use what you've learned to do a little cognitive-behavioral work on yourself. What are your worst fears? Do you worry about the burden you bear for your loved one's diet or restrictions? Are you petrified by the prospect of your loved one's death or disability at an early age? How about problems dealing with the pain and anger and depression your loved one might feel? All of these are sources of fear I often hear expressed.

June and Barbara: Once you've identified these fears, what do you do about them?

Dr. Rubin: It certainly makes sense to talk about them with your diabetic loved one, though you need to find a way to do this that doesn't sound like an attack. The key is to make it clear that these are *your* fears, and that you're not blaming your loved one for them. You can, for example, make statements like, "I get really scared when you have a bad reaction," or "I feel helpless when you get depressed over your diabetes," or "Sometimes I have nightmares about you going on dialysis." Sometimes it helps just to get these feelings of fear off your chest.

Other times you might want to work out a better way of dealing with your fears besides just giving voice to them. You and your loved one could do this together. You could ask if there's anything you could do to help when the diabetic person seems depressed, for instance. If there was something you could do, you'd probably feel less helpless and afraid. But keep in mind that there's not always something you *can* do. In fact, some of your fears may stem in part from your understandable wish to control the uncontrollable.

If your fears persist, you might think about joining a support group where you can talk with other people in the same boat. This could help a lot. Finally, if your fears are really getting out of hand and you are having serious problems coping with them, think about getting some counseling. Remember, you're living with diabetes, too, and you deserve all the help you can get.

June and Barbara: However you get there, when you finally feel calm and less fearful in your own heart and mind, what are some of the ways to transfer these new confident feelings to the diabetic?

Dr. Rubin: In a nutshell, you need to help your loved one find his or her own way through the fears you've just negotiated. That's not to say that your fears and those of your loved one will be identical, but I've found that they're often related. Usually when they aren't the same, they are the flip side of the same coin. As an example of this, you may be afraid that your loved one is ignoring his or her disease; your loved one may be afraid that his or her whole life may be consumed by it.

Actually, once you've confronted your own fears, you will probably already be actively engaged in helping your loved one confront his or hers. That's because you've started talking with each other. Try to continue this process. Trade stories about fears, talk about ways you might help each other. You each have your own fears, but you're in the same boat. Hold each other, love each other, have some fun together. Go to a support group meeting together. Go to a good diabetes education program together. At the Johns Hopkins Diabetes Center where I work, we strongly encourage diabetic participants to bring a loved one. I never cease to be amazed at the benefits couples gain when they spend a week together at the Center. They learn a lot about diabetes, about themselves, and about each other. They leave so much happier, stronger, and less afraid than when they arrived. It's a joy to see the transformation.

➤

FRUSTRATION
IT'S NO MYTH FOR A DIABETIC

Mythological stories of gods and demigods often allegorically illustrate phenomena we encounter in our daily lives. One example is a diabetic's constant emotional companion: frustration. The lead characters in several myths experienced this emotion in the extreme.

Take, for example, two who were condemned to eternal torture. One was Sisyphus, the King of Corinth. Because of his disrespect for Zeus, he was sent to Tartarus, the lowest level of hell. There it was his lot to have to push a heavy rock up a steep hill. Just as it would reach the top, it would slip from his fingers and roll back down. He had to push it up again. It rolled down again. This went on forever, just as your daily uphill push of your heavy diabetes responsibilities goes on forever. Frustrating!

The second was Tantalus, the son of Zeus. Because his insolent behavior roused his father's ire, Zeus also sent him to Tartarus. (Vindictive old coot, wasn't he?) In Tartarus, poor Tantalus was afflicted with hunger and thirst. He was constantly *tantalized* by having food and drink displayed before him, but every time he tried to eat the fruit or drink the waters they receded to just beyond his reach. How's this for a vivid illustration of the frustration of staying on the diabetic diet?

Then there is a more modern frustration myth. Back in the politically incorrect 40s or 50s, a series of "Little Moron" stories circulated. Here's a particularly popular one: Question: Why did the Little Moron beat his head against a stone wall? Answer: Because it felt so good when he stopped.

You aren't as lucky as the legendary Little Moron. You never get to stop. You have to keep eternally beating your head against the stone wall of trying to keep your blood sugars normal. What have you done to deserve this? Nothing! You're a fairly intelligent person, certainly no moron, and you can't have displeased Zeus. You've never even *met* Zeus! But here you are stuck with eternal frustration.

Since you can't ever totally get rid of it, you have to learn to diminish as much of it as you can, and learn to live with the rest. Dr. Rubin has his work cut out for him here!

—June and Barbara

June and Barbara: What are some of the most common frustrations your patients tell you about in connection with diabetes?

Dr. Rubin: When you have diabetes, there's a lot to feel frustrated about. Here are the ones I hear about the most:

1. People feel frustrated that they have to keep their diabetes in mind every waking hour, 365 days a year (366 days in leap year, as an 8-year-old patient once reminded me). A man said to me, "I've had diabetes for 20 years and not a day passes that I don't want to take the diabetes out of me and shoot it." Often the frustration comes from feeling that diabetes limits freedom, freedom to go out and unselfconsciously have fun, for example. A woman told me she had been traveling a lot, including many social meals. This left her frustrated on the one hand

when she had to curtail her eating and frustrated on the other when she *had* to eat to treat low blood sugar.

2. Another source of frustration is the ignorance, insensitivity, or overprotective attitude of other people regarding diabetes and its treatment.

3. People are also often frustrated by the relatively slow progress of medical science in its efforts to develop a preventive or cure for diabetes. Needless to say, this frustration is shared by many doctors and researchers in the field. One colleague of mine told me that he had made a slide 10 years ago to illustrate a talk he was giving. The slide read, "A cure in 10 years." Now, a decade later, he related ruefully, he could still use the same slide.

4. Most of all, people are frustrated by the unpredictable nature of their own bodies. There are times when you do everything you've been taught for good control and yet your blood sugars make no sense. These are the most frustrating times of all, and they come to every diabetic all too frequently. Listen to some of the accounts I've heard:

"Sometimes my blood sugar will remain between 55 mg/dl (3.05 mmol/L) and 110 mg/dl (6.1 mmol/L)for several days, then stay between 200 mg/dl (11.1 mmol/L) and 250 mg/dl (13.8 mmol/L) for several days, with no apparent difference in diet and exercise and with insulin increased in an effort to compensate for the higher sugars. This leaves me so frustrated."

"I always eat the same breakfast every morning. On two consecutive days (with no morning exercise) my blood sugar before lunch was 143 mg/dl (7.9 mmol/L) and 163 mg/dl (9.0 mmol/L). On the third day I had a lot of exercise during the morning. My blood sugar before lunch was 325 mg/dl (18.0 mmol/L)."

"Three months after taking a diabetes self-management course and really getting my act together, I went to the doctor for a hemoglobin A_{1c} test. To tell the truth, I was actually looking forward to it, because I was expecting a really good number. When the test came back at 15 percent I was convinced it was wrong and sent for a retest. That came back 14 percent. Naturally, I was dismayed, frustrated, and angry. I just don't see how I could be under such poor control. I've worked really hard to stick to the diet and exercise. I've carefully calculated my insulin doses. And this is what I end up with. It's enough to make me say, 'to hell with it.'"

The following questions deal with how to handle these uncomfortable feelings of frustration.

June and Barbara: In his book *Feeling Good, the New Mood Therapy,* Dr. David Burns says that frustration results from unrealistic expectations. Diabetics, when being trained to control their blood sugar, are often given many positive expectations. Health professionals and literature assure them, "If you do *this*, the result will always be *that*." Naturally, diabetics expect these predictions to be realistic. But are they? In diabetes, *that* doesn't always follow *this*. Most people find that on occasions their blood sugar goes high even when, as they often put it, they "did everything right." The logical extension of the Burns theory is that controlling diabetes is not a realistic expectation. You're bound to be frustrated. Therefore, you should just give up trying, right? Isn't that the way to avoid frustration?

Dr. Rubin: Nice try, Barbara and June, but no way. I agree with Burns that unrealistic expectations lead to frustration, but our goal is to set expectations that are both ambitious and achievable, not to give up altogether.

It might help to talk about what is realistic and what isn't when it comes to diabetes self-care. Perfection is not realistic. Expecting to get the same blood-sugar result every time your regimen is the same is not realistic. On the other hand, good control is realistic. So is the expectation that *most* of the time you will get a *similar* blood-sugar result if you eat the same, exercise the same, and medicate yourself the same.

This reminds me of Lawrence Pray's book, *Journey of a Diabetic*. Pray has had diabetes since he was a child, for about 40 years. In one passage of his book he advises his fellow diabetics: "Don't try to be perfect. Try for good control, to be sure. But perfection lasts for a moment, and diabetes lasts a lifetime." Wise words. I take them to mean that if you are in for the long haul, which you must be if you have diabetes, you must adopt an attitude that will sustain you throughout your efforts. Perfectionism is not a viable long-haul attitude, because it cannot be successfully sustained. When you're less than perfect, which is inevitable, much of the time you may feel so frustrated that you say, To hell with it.

The two extremes—being a perfectionist versus giving up—often go hand-in-hand as two phases of a cycle that a person tends to repeat. Listen to this man: "I've had diabetes for 36 years, and my pattern has been the same the whole time. I go through a period where I try to achieve really tight control, and I get a lot of lows. Then I say to hell with it, and I binge for a couple of days. This makes me feel terrible physically and emotionally, and I get back on track and start the cycle all over again."

June and Barbara: Imagine repeating that cycle for 36 years! That seems a very long time to frustrate yourself first in one direction and then in another. Is there no cure for this kind of behavior?

Dr. Rubin: The key is not to get stuck, as this man was, in this kind of hopeless process. If you're faced with a blood sugar or series of blood sugars—low or high—that make no sense at all to you, don't let yourself stew. Instead, brainstorm with someone else (another diabetic, someone you're close to, or a member of your health-care team). Two heads are better than one. It's not essential that you actually figure out what's causing the seemingly inexplicable blood sugars, since that will often be impossible. What really matters is that you not feel so frustrated that you give up taking care of yourself. I've found that people don't give up if they can accept the fact that there are times (fortunately, not most of the time) when a blood-sugar reading will simply make no sense. Just deal with it and move on.

June and Barbara: That is so true. It took June years to come to this conclusion and stop fretting about the times when she couldn't make head or tails out of her meter readings. Sometimes her blood sugars are abnormally high for an entire week, and then eventually return to what she considers her usual level. All she does is increase her insulin dosage until diabetes settles down again and she can go back to her normal dosage until the high part of the cycle repeats itself, as it invariably does. So, as you say, just deal with it and move on.

We've been discussing the frustration of trying to be a perfectionist with blood sugars, but what about all the other frustrations of handling life with diabetes?

Dr. Rubin: My philosophy is that in general what you need to do when feeling frustrated is to work smarter rather than harder. The people who tend to feel least frustrated by the never-ending, unyielding facts of life with diabetes are those who make the routine as easy for themselves as possible. Try to think of the times you feel most frustrated. What are the bottlenecks or major hassles in your regimen? Perhaps one of your biggest frustrations is getting the exercise you want; or maybe it's finding yourself somewhere without your insulin and therefore unable to join your friends in enjoying a meal; or maybe you eat out a lot and you always end up torn between feeling deprived and feeling guilty.

Any of these situations can trigger frustration. The key to making each of them easier and less troublesome is the same: plan ahead. In these situations an ounce of prevention is truly worth a ton of cure. Let's take the exercise frustration. If you want to make this as easy as possible, you need to think of the kind of exercise you like best, the amount you want to do, the most convenient time to do it, and the things you need to set up to make exercise happen with the fewest possible hitches.

I love to run, and it's the perfect exercise for me, because I can do it in bits of time, whenever those bits are available. If I have 45 minutes, I can be in my running gear, out the door, finish my run, shower, and be ready for whatever comes next. Some of you might prefer a social setting like a gym or club for your exercise. If you want to go there regularly and this doesn't happen naturally, you need to make it easier for yourself. You might keep the gear in the car and go right after work, to pick one possibility. The point is not the specific solution but the general one. You need to operate like one of those little wind-up cars that backs up and goes in another direction when it hits an obstacle. It's okay to say that one thing won't work and another won't work, as long as you keep asking yourself what *might* work until you find something that does.

Eating out is another potentially frustrating situation. Again, the key to making it easier is planning. You need to decide on what you want to eat before you set foot inside the restaurant. I don't mean you need to have the exact menu in mind, but you need to think about whether you're going to skip the soup and have the bread, or choose a main dish without sauce and go for the dessert. There are no right or wrong choices for any given occasion. I'm just suggesting realistic expectations here. If you go in without a plan, you set yourself up for frustration. Each choice you make will feel like a struggle. If you go in with a plan in mind, you'll find it much easier and more pleasant. At least, that's what I hear from almost everyone I know who tries this preplanning approach. You take the pressure off yourself emotionally, which keeps you from feeling overwhelmingly frustrated.

Admittedly, there are going to be situations you can't plan for. How do you make it easy on yourself under those conditions? Basically, the approach is similar: get your expectations in line with reality and the pressure will go down a lot. You need to take off as much pressure as possible so that you won't break down. You want to maintain your strength and your confidence. The strategies we've just discussed allow you to do that.

June and Barbara: One of the highest levels of frustration comes when an illness—the flu, surgery, or even a simple cold—sends blood sugar sky-high and there seems to be no way to bring it down. Should one accept this out-of-control situation and just say, "This, too, shall pass?"

Dr. Rubin: Actually, the attitude you suggest is a fairly constructive one, but more on this later. Let's first analyze what's happening here. An illness is a stress upon the body. Your body becomes stressed to a degree that throws you completely out of whack. This has a frustratingly destabilizing effect on blood sugars, even when everything else is stable. This same kind of out-of-whackness can be caused just as well by emotional stress as by physiological stress. We'll talk about physical stress first, then emotional, and then ways to handle either kind.

Illness is one of the most frustrating situations for people with diabetes. As one man put it, "Diabetes has a mind of its own. If you get an infection, no matter how well you've been doing before, it all goes out the window." When you're sick, the whole carefully constructed edifice of your diabetes regimen collapses like a house of cards. You can't exercise, you don't feel like eating, and the infection itself seems to play havoc with your insulin needs. (Type II's may have to temporarily take insulin injections during illness.) Taken together, what you have is your basic mess. And it's such an unpredictable mess. While most people find that illness pushes their blood sugars through the roof, some have the opposite problem. One woman said, "When I get sick, I have no appetite at all. Since I'm diabetic, I have to force myself to eat. But even though I cut way back on my insulin, I still end up with lots of reactions. It feels horrible, and I get so frustrated."

Even if you usually go high when you're sick, as most people do, reactions can be a problem. You can overshoot with insulin as you try to bring down a high blood sugar, especially if you have ketones, and you *have* to clear them. (Ketones are the poisonous acid by-products of your body's desperate efforts to sustain itself by burning fat when you don't have enough insulin in your system.) Some of my most frustrating moments were times when my son was sick and we were pumping him with insulin because of ketones. There he was with a low blood sugar, ketones, and feeling so nauseous that he could hardly hold down anything. We had to give him insulin to get rid of those damned ketones, but we also had to get him to eat or drink something to avoid a horrible reaction. Somehow, we survived. Flat Coke was usually the key to managing these moments.

I should mention here that stress-induced high blood sugars can come from other sources, such as premenstrual syndrome, or from drugs like prednisone, which one of my patients had to take to sustain her transplanted liver and kidney.

June and Barbara: Most of us can see fairly easily how physical stress can interfere with blood sugar, but at least after an illness or surgery the diabetic person can resume the regular regimen and settle down again. Most of us find mental or emotional stress a much more mysterious thing and harder to even recognize, as it can come on instantly and disappear fast or it can hang around and become more or less chronic.

Dr. Rubin: Let me give you a classic example of the power of emotional stress. This is an experience I had with my son Stefan four years ago when he turned 16. We were getting ready to head over to the Motor Vehicle Administration for his driver's test. He wisely decided to check his blood sugar before we left, because he wanted to avoid being either too high or too low and thus risk a poor performance on the test. He found he was about 140 mg/dl (7.7 mmol/L), which seemed just fine, so off we went.

Unfortunately, luck was not with us that day, and Stefan failed the test. When we got back home, less than an hour after we had left, he complained that he was feeling high. We tested and found that he was over 400 mg/dl (22.2 mmol/L). And this without any food over the previous several hours.

A week later Stefan was ready for another driver's test, though I really wasn't. Once again he checked his blood sugar before leaving and once again he was just under 140 mg/dl (7.7 mmol/L). This time he passed the test. When we got home, he said he was feeling fine and was eager to go out and make use of his new driving privilege. I, ever the Sympathetic (but exigent) Scientist, insisted that he test his blood again. It was 240 mg/dl (13.3 mmol/L). My theory is that he was under stress both times he took the driving test. This pushed his blood sugar up some. The first time the stress continued after he failed the test as he contemplated his fate, and this pushed his sugar up even more. The second time, once he passed the test, his blood sugar leveled off.

June and Barbara: What should you do when your body is stressed physically or emotionally and your blood sugars go crazy in unfamiliar and frustrating ways?

Dr. Rubin: First, understand that this does happen. I'm still amazed to find people who have never been told this. One man told me that he couldn't understand why he couldn't get his blood sugars under control when he was sick. Only later, after much frustration, fear, and self-castigation, did his doctor tell him, "This is normal, and you shouldn't worry about it."

Second, repeat to yourself, as many times as you need to, the following words: "This is not my fault." You're so used to having things go at least fairly predictably when you do the right (or even wrong) thing, it's hard to accept it could be otherwise when you're sick or under pressure. Feeling frustrated and worried only makes matters worse, but it's almost instinctive. As one of my patients said, "I feel as though I'm doing something wrong, and I go over and over the list of possibilities.

Have I eaten too much? I know I haven't exercised, could that be it? Everyone says it's just what happens when you get an infection, and I know in my head they are right. But I still feel kind of out of control and really frustrated with myself." This man definitely needs to repeat to himself, "This is not my fault." He needs to kick out the Pushy Prosecutor and call in the Sympathetic Scientist.

Third, you can take some steps to restabilize yourself as quickly as possible. The keys are testing, adjusting, and getting advice and counsel, if you need them. When you're sick, it's important to test frequently especially if you're prone to ketones, as most Type I's are. You can't know for sure you have ketones unless you test your urine (using Chemstrips UGK or Ketostix). Sometimes you may suspect you have ketones because you feel really rotten and sick to your stomach. If you do find ketones in your urine, you should get in touch with your doctor for advice on how to adjust your insulin to get rid of them. You'll also need to increase the frequency of your blood tests. It's like flying when the weather is stormy and the visibility poor; you want all the information you can get from the instruments available. Getting your blood sugars restabilized will make you feel better physically and will set your mind at ease, as well.

Sometimes, through some combination of emotional and physical wackiness, you may find yourself unable to make the best decisions for yourself when sick or under emotional stress. If so, get help. Call on any family member who knows enough about diabetes to give good advice, or a diabetic friend, or, of course, the medical staff who treat you. Don't hesitate to call the doctor or nurse. That's what they're there for. They would much rather help you manage your problem at home than treat you in the emergency room later. I'm not suggesting that any of these people will have *the* answer, but talking to them can provide relief and some useful suggestions.

Finally we come back to the solution you offered in your question. Yes, I think it's a good idea to tell yourself, "This, too, shall pass." This horrible, rotten, no good, very bad feeling will not go on forever, though you might feel as if it will when you're in the middle of it. Just take it one step and one test at a time. Keep doing what you should, in consultation with people you trust to advise you, and it will pass.

June and Barbara: We've heard a lot of complaints about health providers and the great frustration they can cause their diabetic patients. For instance, "He won't talk to me." "She never returns my calls." "Over the 22 years I've lived with diabetes, I have never seen a doctor who truly understands what it's like to live with a chronic illness."

On the opposite side of the coin, we've heard equally as many complaints from nurses and doctors about the behavior of diabetics. "He simply won't exercise." "She hasn't lost a single pound in six months." "Frank is in the hospital again with ketoacidosis."

Dr. Rubin: This is a common problem. Its source, as with any frustration, is disappointed expectations. Let's look first at the expectations diabetics have of health professionals. Some diabetics simply want to be "fixed." They're looking for doctor to perform some sort of medical magic and leave them with normal blood sugars or, at least, the ability to create that result on their own. Another related expectation I often hear expressed is that the doctor be completely knowledgeable, up-to-date on the latest technology, and infallible in explaining every erstwhile (often inexplicable) diabetes-related occurrence in their lives. On the emotional level, diabetics want their doctors to be "human," available when needed, understanding, compassionate, attentive, and unhurried. Finally, many diabetics wish, even if they don't expect it, that their doctors would really understand what it's like (read: how hard it is) to have diabetes.

What about the doctor's expectations? He or she expects the diabetic to be motivated, to *want* to achieve and maintain good control, and to follow advice designed to produce that outcome. The doctor also expects that good control will inevitably follow good self-care, even as day follows night. When doctors see that a patient isn't sticking to the regimen, they almost always attribute this failing to a lack of motivation. One interesting study compared reasons that doctors cited for their diabetic patients' dietary noncompliance, and reasons diabetics gave for this same behavior. Eighty percent of the doctors attributed non-compliance primarily to lack of motivation, and 10 percent to patients' lack of information. In contrast, only 34 percent of the patients named lack of motivation as the principal cause of their dietary problems, and only 2 percent named lack of information. Patients were much more likely to point to environmental factors (life circumstances such as family, job, or economic conditions) or physical limitations such as visual handicaps or limited mobility that interfered with food preparation. Thirty-eight percent of the diabetics said that environmental factors were the primary obstacle, and 26 percent said that physical limitations were the principal problem. Doctors never mentioned either of these causes.

My point in citing the findings of this study is not to suggest that the patients were right and the doctors wrong or the opposite. Instead, I think these data reflect the wide gap between the views each group holds of the problems they are joined in trying to solve. These views inevitably lead to divergent and unrealistic expectations, the perfect setup for frustration. Each expects the other to be more than he or she can realistically be. Not that these expectations make no sense. Diabetes is a serious matter. Each party genuinely wants a good result and tries hard to get that result. Each also feels deeply disappointed when that result is not forthcoming. That frustration is often directed inward ("I must have done something wrong"). But, since we are all human, we naturally direct some of that frustration outward as well.

June and Barbara: Directing it outward explains why we have heard so many complaints from both doctors and diabetics about the failures of the other party. How can both groups come to terms with their feelings about one another?

Dr. Rubin: To manage these uncomfortable and usually wasteful feelings you must:

➤ Accept that these feelings are natural, normal, even inevitable.
➤ Understand that their source is disappointed expectations.
➤ Identify those expectations that have been disappointed.
➤ Decide which of these expectations are realistic and which are not.

In general, speaking on the doctors' side, I have found that if I expect all my patients to be highly motivated, my expectation is unrealistic and I'm sure to feel frustrated in many cases. I need to accept that some people who consult me are not motivated. I also need to accept that to expect I can motivate them is equally unrealistic. I wish I had that kind of power, but I don't. I can only help people find their own motivation. This is a very important distinction, because my job is then defined in realistic terms and so are my patients'. This allows us to get down to the business of doing those jobs without setting ourselves up for disappointment and frustration.

This reminds me of a story I read a couple of years ago. A woman had been going to a wonderful, if somewhat traditional, doctor for years. The physician retired and turned his practice over to a younger man. The woman sat in the waiting room on her first appointment with the new doctor. He approached her and introduced himself as her "junior partner in health care." The message was clear: this was a partnership, and his role was essential but was clearly a secondary, facilitative one, not that of the all-knowing, all-powerful final authority on all things medical.

June and Barbara: What a refreshing attitude on the part of the doctor!

Dr. Rubin: Either party can bring this kind of reality to the doctor-patient relationship. You need to recognize and accept what your doctor can do and what is beyond his or her power, and you need a physician who will work with you on this kind of realistic partnership. Remember, having realistic expectations of your doctor doesn't mean having no expectations at all, or feeling that the whole burden for your care is yours alone. Many of the expectations you have for your health-care provider are probably quite realistic. You need to work with the doctor to see that you get what you deserve—whether that may be the time to ask questions or get full answers to the questions you ask, or an honest, open, compassionate attitude, or any specific services you feel you need.

➤ Help for Those Who Want to Help Diabetics

June and Barbara: Jean-Paul Sartre said that "Hell is other people." Sometimes we think that could be amended to read "diabetic other people." We see those who are close to diabetics put through manifold hells of frustration when their loved ones don't or won't take care of their disease. How can these frustrated significant others accept or combat those feelings without getting all riled up or being mean to the diabetic who is causing that frustration?

Dr. Rubin: Other people never cause frustration or any other feeling, good or bad. I'm happy to make this point once again, because it's so important yet rarely understood. No one can *cause* you to feel anything or do anything. All they can do is "push your button," as the popular phrase goes. They can trigger a feeling you already have. If there's no feeling there, no button to be pushed, all the effort in the world can't cause you to feel it.

No doubt you'll feel plenty if someone pushes a sensitive button. Here's an example. Terri feels overwhelmingly frustrated by her diabetic mother's attitude toward self-care. The younger woman said to me, "Whenever I try to help her, she just says, 'If I go blind, I go blind.' It drives me crazy." Is Terri's mother driving her crazy? Most of you would probably say yes, but I'd suggest otherwise.

What's driving Terri crazy is not the fact her mother doesn't care if she goes blind, but the fact that Terri's own expectations are being disappointed. She thinks her mother *should* care about going blind, and that she *should* be able to lead her mother in the paths of diabetic righteousness. This might sound like an unimportant distinction, even a purely semantic one, but it's actually a critical distinction. Her mother isn't causing the frustration Terri feels. Her own disappointed expectations are. To make this point, let's imagine how Terri would feel if it were someone other than her mother who expressed these fatalistic thoughts—the mother of an associate at work, for instance. Would this make Terri feel crazy with frustration? Almost certainly not. Her feeling would more likely be pity, or sympathy, or wonder. The specific feeling we have and how intensely we feel it depends on us, on our expectations, not on the behavior that triggers the feeling.

June and Barbara: Yes, but how does the daughter go about feeling less crazy and avoid letting her mother push her crazy-frustration button? This routine has probably been going on a long time between mother and daughter and is nicely established by now.

Dr. Rubin: Terri has to find a way to deactivate the button herself. Here's how she can do it step by step:

> 1. She must identify the disappointed expectations that are driving her crazy. They seem to be the expectation that her mother will care about going blind, and the expectation that Terri can make her mother care.
>
> 2. Next Terri needs to ask herself whether these expectations are realistic. In this case, the proof of the pudding is that they aren't. For some other person or some other situation they might be. In the best of all possible worlds they would be. But that's not the point.

The point is here and now, and here and now these are unrealistic expectations.

3. Next Terri must grieve her failed expectations. She has to feel angry, depressed, and ultimately accepting of the fact that these hopes will not be realized. This is hard and takes time, but it must be done.

4. Finally, she must find another attitude and approach to her mother, one based on realistic expectations. This attitude might be something like this: "I love my mother, and I'll do my best to help her see the light, but I can't make her do the right thing. I have to accept my limits. Once I've done what I can, I have to let go, hard as this is for me when I see what she's doing to herself."

June and Barbara: That's really tough to do. It's terrible to stand by and watch a loved one go blind.

Dr. Rubin: It's really the only way to go. It protects you from going crazy, it protects your relationship with the other person, and it might even improve chances for the other person to do what you wanted in the first place. To understand what I mean by the last, listen to a diabetic man I spoke to recently: "Everyone in my family is always telling me what I should and shouldn't do, even my grandchildren. I guess what I really need to do is to stop getting so frustrated with them and become more familiar with my friend diabetes." Bingo! Once this man accepts that the frustration he feels is within him and not with his family, he can turn his energy toward "getting more familiar with his friend diabetes." Something similar might happen for Terri's mother. If Terri stopped pushing so hard, her mother might stop using all of her energy pushing back, and she might have a little left for taking care of herself.

June and Barbara: Even if you solve your frustration problems with the diabetic, you're still left with the problem of trying to help alleviate the diabetic's frustration with the disease.

Of course, the first step in doing that is to have a thorough understanding of the disease and the diabetic's personal regimen, so you'll know what he or she is supposed to be doing.

The second, and more difficult, step is to gain empathy with the diabetic's frustration—to feel how it really feels. One way to do this is to pretend to be diabetic yourself for a few weeks. We first heard about this idea from a diabetes program in an Australian hospital. There they made the staff members live as if they were diabetic: take shots (of saline solution), test their blood sugar several times a day, rigidly follow the diabetic diet, get the right amount of exercise, always be sure to have snacks on hand—and eat them even when they didn't feel like eating. These staff members quickly got the picture that handling diabetes wasn't as easy as it might appear, or as easy as they frequently made it sound when they gave instruction to patients.

Barbara tried this game of "Let's Pretend," except that she shot up vitamin B instead of saline. Despite the fact that she thought she already knew everything there was to know about what a diabetic has to go through on a daily basis, she gained a new perspective when she had to do it herself. You might try this empathy exercise yourself.

Still, even pretending to be a diabetic doesn't give you the total picture. It may show you how frustrating it is to try to fit all the time-consuming, mind-preoccupying, inexorable diabetes routines into your life, but it can't let you experience what it's like when you've done everything exactly the way you're supposed to and it doesn't work and you can't decide what to do next.

One thing Barbara sometimes does—although not voluntarily—is to make that decision. On those occasions when June has reached her apogee of frustration, and Barbara is standing on the periphery asking questions and muttering suggestions, June has been known to blow an exasperation gasket and say, "I don't know what to do. I admit it. You're such a great diabetes expert and have so many brilliant ideas, you tell me exactly what I should do and I'll do it."

At this Barbara gulps, squares her shoulders, and delivers herself of a wise decision (translation: she makes an educated guess). About half the time it works. Since that's approximately how June's own "wise decisions" usually work out, Barbara feels she's done no harm. (Hippocratic Oath: First, do no harm.) At least she's shared some of the burden of frustration for a little while. On top of that, she really understands what that burden feels like when it's on her own back.

Dr. Rubin, how do family members or friends of your patients come up with effective schemes to alleviate the diabetic's frustration?

Dr. Rubin: The key to developing effective frustration reduction schemes is trial and error. Here are some hints for your trials that might minimize your errors.

Diabetics who are overwhelmed by frustration need support. Support comes in two forms: emotional and practical, and both are effective when you've had it up to here with the daily hassles of living with diabetes. I can't tell you how many times a diabetic has said to me something like this: "I was just feeling beside myself last night when my meter read 367. Then my wife put her arms around me and gave me a big hug. It didn't lower my blood sugar, but it certainly raised my spirits." Just knowing you are not alone can work wonders. So try saying to your diabetic loved one, "I love you. I will do anything I can to help. I know there's only so much I can do, but let me hold you and listen to you."

Practical support is also much appreciated by most diabetics. You can help alleviate frustration by taking on any diabetes-related chores that burden your loved one and that you feel you can handle.

June and Barbara: We know for a fact that even the smallest chore-handling can make a big difference. For example, if you always carry glucose tablets and snacks for the diabetic, it will not only help alleviate the frustration he or she feels when the snack pack runs dry and there's nothing around to eat, but it will give the diabetic a great feeling of security to know that someone else is ready to help out in an emergency.

Knowing how to give a shot is also important, even if you're hardly ever asked to do it. In the beginning June often welcomed having Barbara give her an injection, but now the only time she asks is when it's difficult for her to reach the injection site—for example, on a plane.

If you have a thorough understanding of the diet your diabetic family member or friend is supposed to follow, you can be of help when it turns out to be a frustrating challenge to piece together an appropriate meal from a strange restaurant menu. One thing Barbara sometimes does: if she sees that June is ordering the dead wrong thing, Barbara will order a diabetically appropriate meal and then offer to trade or share when the food arrives and June clearly sees the error of her order.

We once reported that little restaurant sleight-of-food trick in a diabetes magazine article. In the next month's Letters to the Editor column we got unholy hell from one reader. She objected that ordering back-up meals like that would be treating diabetics like idiots and coddling them and that they should be free to make their own mistakes and live with them and learn from them. So, it seems that even in well-intentioned frustration-alleviation techniques, one diabetic's meat can be another's poison.

Dr. Rubin: Yes, you always have to personalize any general guidelines for helping a diabetic. Communication is at the heart of this process. If you're in a situation where you want to help and you're not sure how to, or if you don't know if what you have in mind to do will be well-received, just ask. A simple, "What can I do to help?" delivered in a loving tone often does the trick. Or, if it seems more appropriate, offer some suggestions, but be sure you keep them in question form: "Are you feeling a little low? Think we should stop for a snack since we're still a long way from home?"

June and Barbara: What if it's not just a one-shot frustration fix? What if you see a pattern of frustration in the diabetic's life, a continuing situation that may need quite a bit of analysis and work to fix?

Dr. Rubin: This does take a different approach. At some quiet, peaceful time when you're both feeling fairly relaxed (don't laugh, these times do come to us all, at least occasionally), talk about what you've noticed. Maybe something like, "It seems that you've been feeling really frustrated with the whole food thing recently. You say you're bored with the meals, and you eat things you say you shouldn't and then you get a major case of the guilts. I love you and hate to see you suffer. Can you think of anything I can do to help?"

If the answer is yes, you're in business. Start brainstorming. If your loved one is open to help but can't think of what you could do, try offering a few suggestions. Remember to cast these suggestions as questions. Ask if you might cook some new and different meals—or cook some meals, period, if you usually don't. One woman told me she and her diabetic husband get a terrific kick out of serving diabetically correct meals at dinner parties, without identifying them as such, and hearing their guests rave. Or you might ask if you should clear the house of junk food, if that seems to be causing a problem.

June and Barbara: This last shows the truth about what you said about personalizing the help you offer. We know some diabetics who build up a huge frustration if there's no candy in the house. It gets so bad that they finally crack and go eat a whole box of chocolates. These same people, if they know there's a box of dietetic chocolates on the shelf and that they can have one—just one—when the pressure gets too strong, can get along quite nicely. For others, if some food is in the house they'll eat it but if it's not there they tend to forget about it. So offering to throw away the junk for them would be a good idea.

But what if your diabetic loved one isn't receptive to any of your help overtures and flatly turns down every suggestion you make?

Dr. Rubin: Don't despair, and try not to get frustrated yourself. Just make sure that the diabetic knows your offer stands, and check back from time to time. Even though this approach sometimes takes a little while to work, it's almost always successful.

One last suggestion. Keep in mind that to reduce your diabetic loved one's frustration, you must address his or her agenda, not yours. Dealing with your loved one's agenda is supportive; dealing with yours is pushing. If *you* decide what's good for your diabetic loved one (unless you've been explicitly asked to do so or you're dealing with an emergency), you may well increase frustration, not reduce it.

CHAPTER 8

GUILT
THE THREE LITTLE GUILT TRIPS

In working with diabetics, we've noticed three different ways to get to the Land of Guilt.

Route No. 1: This is exemplified by an article we once read in *Ski* magazine, a story about the McCoy family of Mammoth Mountain, California. The father, Dave, founded and developed the giant ski resort area. He was also well known as a coach of the U.S. ski team, of which his daughter, Penny, was a member. This is how she described his coaching methods:

> As a coach, Dad was as inspiring as he was a great technician. Once I came down and I thought I skied terribly. I was really upset.
> When he asked what was bothering me I told him and he said, "Okay, what did you do right? I want you to go back up and think about nothing else except what you did right."

Of course, her next run was much better. As she said, "That taught me to think about things I can do and not about things I can't do."

Diabetics who take the "I did everything wrong" approach to guilt are those who sincerely try hard to keep in control and when they make any mistake they beat themselves over the head with a guilt cudgel, never thinking of how well they generally do, never giving themselves credit for their almost-always-successful diabetes self-therapy.

Route No. 2: This is described in a small book we once read, a kind of fable for people who are trying to lose weight. In this story a little overweight bear felt bad about being fat. She felt so bad about it that she had to eat for solace. That, of course made her feel even worse, so she ate still more, which made her feel terrible, so she . . . well, you get the picture. (The story had a happy ending when she found a friend who helped her gain the self-esteem needed to lose weight.)

This fable shows how some diabetics—often those in the same weight-problem situation as the bear—break their diet or don't exercise and then feel so guilty about it that they do more of the same to try to make themselves feel better.

Route No. 3: This is the one taken by Isadora Wing, the heroine in Erica Jong's novels *Fear of Flying* and *How to Save Your Own Life*. It was Isadora's method of operation to do exactly what she wanted to and then feel guilty about it.

This is a popular route for diabetics. It makes guilt the price you pay for your transgressions. If you feel really guilty, you've paid a high enough price to completely absolve yourself. Then you feel free to "go thou and sin some more."

These are the three main routes for guilt trips. Whichever one you generally take to the Land of Guilt—or even if, like the Stephen Leacock character, you fling yourself upon your horse and ride off madly in all directions—Dr. Rubin will help you change your course so you'll wind up in a better and happier place.

—June and Barbara

June and Barbara: Guilt and shame are terms that people, including us, sometimes confuse. Could you differentiate between guilt and shame for us? Are diabetics more likely to experience one rather than the other (or both simultaneously)?

Dr. Rubin: I've always made this distinction between guilt and shame: guilt is what you feel when you do something bad; shame is what you feel when someone sees you do it. You might feel guilty if you eat something you shouldn't, and ashamed if your spouse walks in and catches you in the act. Since we commit most of our transgressions without an audience, guilt is a more common feeling than shame.

By the very nature of these two definitions, you can't feel ashamed unless you feel guilty first. If you overeat, don't test your blood sugar, don't exercise, or forget your oral medication, you feel guilty. You'll only feel ashamed if someone who knows what you should be doing finds out about your lapses. For all of us shame is particularly painful, because it's a kind of double-whammy. It's that awful feeling of having our sins exposed for all to see.

June and Barbara: We hear so much these days about being responsible for our own health and even bringing on disease because of our mental attitude (for example, Type A personalities being likely to get heart attacks, depressed people who let others rule their lives being likely to get cancer). Do you find that many of your patients actually feel guilty about having diabetes, feel that they must have done something wrong to bring it on? We've known people who erroneously tortured themselves because they thought they must have eaten too much sugar and that's what caused their diabetes. Others may think their poor mental attitude is the culprit.

Dr. Rubin: I must say that I know very few diabetics who feel responsible for getting the disease. I wonder if people in your state of California are more likely to believe that their minds have a profound effect on their bodies. The fact is that no one knows exactly what causes diabetes. We're only sure of one thing: there is a genetic factor, and none of us should feel responsible for the set of genes we're born with.

I do find that people think a lot about what caused their diabetes, and many of them believe stress played a major role.

Some folks mention that they were diagnosed after a particularly difficult period of caring for a terminally ill spouse or parent. Others recall a car accident or a work-related injury that immediately preceded their diagnosis. Still others will cite some major emotional upheaval like losing a job or relocating.

June and Barbara: Beware of talk about car accidents causing diabetes! In one of our previous books we mentioned that the stress of an automobile accident could bring on diabetes, and ever since we've been plagued by letters and calls from lawyers trying to prove their clients' diabetes was caused by an automobile accident. Unfortunately for them, we could not report any specific incidents that could be used in court.

When we asked diabetes experts Richard Guthrie, M.D., and Diana Guthrie, R.N., Ph.D., they had no specifics to report, either. In fact Richard Guthrie was of the opinion that some of the people who thought their diabetes was brought on by an accident actually may have already had diabetes but it was not diagnosed until they were in the hospital as a result of the accident.

Dr. Rubin: I agree that where diabetes is concerned, people sometimes fall victim to post hoc reasoning—the erroneous belief that because something happened just before the diagnosis, it caused the diabetes. One of the best stories I've heard about stress causing diabetes was this one, told to me a few years ago by a woman in a group I was leading: "One morning I was sitting down to my breakfast, and this huge spider plopped down on the table right in front of my face. I was so upset I almost had a heart attack. And the next week I got diabetes. I know it was that spider that did it. I've always been deathly afraid of them."

It's easy to laugh at the idea that the spider who sat down beside her caused this lady's diabetes. But before we laugh too loudly, we should remember that stress can affect people's blood-sugar levels once they've gotten diabetes. Is it also possible that stress can push them into diabetes in the first place?

Some of the most advanced thinking suggests that getting diabetes is like turning a key in a lock. To work, the key has to line up with each of the tumblers inside the lock. Similarly, to get diabetes a combination of factors—environmental, genetic, and cellular—must all line up. Stress could well be one of the environmental factors. It could provide the final push that overwhelms the insulin-producing beta cells of the pancreas, sort of like the last bit of water that finally bursts the dam.

What I've just described is still pretty speculative. I find theories about the causes of diabetes interesting, whether they come from scientists or from diabetics themselves.

June and Barbara: Getting back to a more narrow interpretation of guilt, here's a perfect example of guilt in action, and it's a word-for-word quotation from a real diabetic: "I know I don't go to the doctor as often as I should, and I know the reason why. I just end up feeling so guilty. She asks me if I've been exercising and I say no. She asks me if I've been testing my blood and I say no. She asks me if I've lost any weight and I say no. She asks me if I've stopped smoking and I say no. With every question I feel worse and worse about myself. She tells me in this really gentle way that there's nothing she can do if I won't help myself, and I know she's right. What's wrong with me?"

What *is* wrong with her?

Dr. Rubin: I guess you mean what's wrong with her for being so helpless and feeling so guilty. The two go hand-in-hand. Guilt can be paralyzing. I talked earlier in the Denial chapter about basic beliefs and automatic thoughts and how powerful they can be in generating either positive or negative emotions and behavior. That's what's going on here as well. When you're guilt-ridden, your basic belief is that you're a bad, weak, self-destructive person incapable of doing anything right, at least when it comes to your diabetes. Springing from this absolutely negative basic belief are specific negative automatic thoughts such as, "I'll never be able to stop smoking," or "I have no will power when it comes to food," or "I'm incapable of losing weight."

June and Barbara: Here's a common specific guilt trigger. We've met a lot of Type II diabetics who feel guilty about being overweight. They know that being overweight exacerbates their diabetes. Their guilt is therefore somewhat valid. Can they in any way use this guilt to good advantage?

Dr. Rubin: Everything I've already said about guilt holds true with this particular problem. Again, to feel guilty and tell yourself you're a bad person and you've done wrong has no advantage. It only saps your strength. But there is a way to shift your thinking into a pattern that will help you lose weight. What you need to do is see the issue as one of accepting responsibility for your actions. Let me explain the difference between these two attitudes. *Feeling guilty* involves negative judgments about yourself, and it focuses on the past in a way that tends to paralyze. *Feeling responsible* involves no judgments, and it focuses on the present and future in a way that tends to motivate.

June and Barbara: How do you go about applying this idea of accepting responsibility if you're an overweight Type II diabetic? It seems to us that it's a long jump from feeling guilty because you haven't accepted responsibility for your weight to actually assuming that responsibility.

Dr. Rubin: The secret is to stay nonjudgmental about yourself and your past failure. You have to focus on the future, not on the past. It works like this. First, you must accept the fact that you *are* responsible for the extra weight you carry. I know there are genetic and other factors involved, but you need to focus on what you can control. You need to accept responsibility for your diet and your exercise program. Think about what changes you could make. If you need to lose lots of weight, you'll probably need to be in a long-term support group. You might succeed on your own, but the odds are against you. The diet has to be one you can live with for the long haul. Crash diets almost never work, and they can create problems for your diabetes, too. Set realistic goals. If you're overly ambitious, you'll end up feeling guilty and discouraged again. One woman I talked with said that her weight-loss goal was 150 pounds, which was a good goal for her. But when I asked her how long she was going to give herself to lose the weight, she said, "Three months." Short of major surgery, that was out of the question.

You must also accept responsibility for the lifestyle changes your weight-loss program will involve. You may end up eating differently from your family and friends, and your social life will almost certainly change. You may need to spend extra time shopping for food and preparing healthy meals. All of these changes can be difficult, and you must be prepared to make them and stick with them if you're to lose weight and keep it off.

June and Barbara: That's a lot of changing, all right, and a lot of self-responsibility. We all agree that diet and weight management are the most difficult aspects of the diabetic regimen, because they're a 24-hour-a-day issue and involve every aspect of personal and social life. It takes incredible strength to make all those changes and have any hope of succeeding. How can you gain this strength?

Dr. Rubin: We're back to avoiding guilt feelings at all costs, because guilt saps your strength. Instead, think about your own personal reasons for losing weight. Keeping them in mind is likely to help you feel constructively responsible. The reasons your doctor or spouse or co-workers give may not be yours. What are yours? Make sure that among these reasons is some positive image of yourself. Each day when you first awaken and just before you go to sleep at night, put that positive image of yourself in your mind and in your heart. This image will carry you in the right direction, guiding you to live each day as self-lovingly as you can.

June and Barbara: Everyone commits a dietary indiscretion occasionally. Some people punish themselves with what seems excessive guilt for such lapses. Is there some good technique to avoiding overreacting to a minor deviation from dietary rules?

Dr. Rubin: Try to identify the thoughts that are triggering your guilty feelings. They'll be unique to you, but here are some I've heard recently that may sound familiar: "Whenever I eat something I shouldn't, I feel like I've ruined my diet." "I binge every night, and then I suffer so, imagining the damage I'm doing to my body. "I have no spine at all. I can't pass the ice cream case in the grocery store without buying something."

Let's say your indiscretions are few and far between, and your guilt is triggered by the belief that any slip ruins your diet. The flaw in this thinking is that you're striving for perfection, which is a worthy goal but unattainable. Psyching out diabetes means finding the easiest way to take good care of yourself, not the hardest. When you grit your teeth and flog yourself onward toward the impossible goal of perfection, you make it harder to achieve a more realistic one. You'll actually get closer to perfection if you appreciate your successes than you will if you minimize them, because motivation is built on a foundation of self-confidence, not self-criticism.

June and Barbara: That sounds logical, but in this case, you've just done something wrong. How are you to build self-confidence on that basis? We'd think you could only get confident as a result of doing things right.

Dr. Rubin: To turn indiscretions into an opportunity to foster self-confidence, you could say to yourself, "I'm feeling guilty, but when I stop to think about it, it's been several days since I slipped. I'm really doing pretty well. No one's perfect." Another version might be, "I was feeling bad (or good), and decided that a treat was what I needed. So I had it. Next time I guess I ought to think what else might have done the trick." The whole point is to give yourself the benefit of another chance and to keep clearly in mind a realistic image of your transgression when viewed in comparison to your overall achievements.

June and Barbara: That's fine for people who have a lapse now and then, but what if your life is pretty much one long series of lapses and you have very few if any positive achievements to keep in mind?

Dr. Rubin: My answer to that is that it only makes it more important for you to find some ways to build your confidence. If your confidence is shaky, it's because your thoughts are negative. Maybe you're stuck with the attitude that you are what you do. The fact that you're doing a bad job with your diet doesn't mean you're a bad person. The key is to reverse your negative thought, because it will only create a negative feeling (guilt), and that will lead to no action. Ask yourself how you might create a mood where something good could happen. Try to see your slips as lessons rather than failures. Changing your perspective this way, if you can do it, will reverse the direction of the thought-feeling-action cycle and turn it positive.

June and Barbara: To understand this clearly, we'd like an example of an actual situation. As one of our editors once told us, "Don't preach. Just show."

Dr. Rubin: Okay, how's this? I had a patient who "grazed" (nibbled pretty much nonstop) every evening between dinner and bedtime. She was convinced that this ruined her diet, so she felt really guilty. She wasn't all that careful about food at other times of the day, either, since she figured her diet was already ruined. We began by working with her thought that the evening grazing ruined her diet. Without much trouble she was able to replace this thought with the thought that she was (or could easily be) doing a good job 20 hours of the day. Right away this eased the guilt and increased her capacity to deal with her vulnerable time.

Then we started working on strategies for dealing with the evening period. She began prepackaging her evening snacks in the morning so she'd be less likely to sit down in front of the television with a whole box of crackers or a whole bag of chips. She started going out more in the evening so she wasn't sitting around feeling bored and empty. She stayed out of the kitchen except when she was having her snack. These positive actions made her feel better and built her self-confidence, just as her more positive thoughts had made her feel better and act more positively. She had activated a positive cycle every bit as powerful and a lot more pleasant than the negative one she'd been living with.

However well or poorly you're doing with your diet, there's room to do better, if you focus on creating a mood where something good can happen. Mobilize, don't paralyze.

June and Barbara: Certain diabetics who are committed to tight control feel guilty when they see a high blood-sugar reading on their meter. They think it's their fault and they start reciting to themselves a long litany of "I should have's." Most of the time these are meaningless, because usually you can't ascertain definitively the cause of a particular high reading. They go on a needless guilt trip. How can they free their minds from this kind of negative routine?

Dr. Rubin: Here's another case where the wisdom of taking responsibility can get confused with the nonsense of feeling guilty. It's wise to recognize that you have a substantial degree of control over your blood-sugar levels. It's also wise to try to figure out why a particular reading is high or low. But, as you point out, it's nonsense to think that you can explain every reading. And, of course, it's damaging to lay a guilt trip on yourself over something that's already happened.

You can approach a high blood-sugar reading wisely if you listen to your Sympathetic Scientist, who would probably say something like this: "So you had a 312. Any idea what might have caused it? Let's see, you had that extra bread at lunchtime, but that wasn't enough to push you up this high. Hmm. Think you might have an infection? No, there's no sign of that. You did miss your exercise, and that might be part of it. You took your morning insulin an hour earlier than usual, too. Maybe that made a difference, though you've done that plenty of times before without going high. Things were pretty stressful at the office. That afternoon meeting made you anxious, and you do go high from stress sometimes. So it could have been the stress, or a little of this and a little of that all put together. Or it could have been just another one of those times, the ones you can't explain no matter how hard you try. Any lessons for the future? Maybe take an extra unit of Regular before stressful meetings, but that's risky, because a reaction in the middle of the meeting is the last thing you want. Maybe test right after the meeting and take the extra insulin then if you're high. That would tell you if it was the stress that pushed up your sugar, and it would let you correct it right away instead of waiting a few hours. Okay, let's think about that for the future. For now, how much extra Regular do you think you should take to get back to normal and put this behind you?"

Unfortunately, most diabetics are more likely to listen to another, louder voice in these situations: the voice of their Pushy Prosecutor. The Prosecutor's approach to a high blood sugar goes like this: "312! Wow! Do you realize how high that is? You must have really screwed up big time to get a 312. All right, I want to know everything you've done since your last test, and don't try to hide anything. You were 128 this morning and now you're 312. An extra bread at lunch, huh? Is that all? It must have been more than that. And you took your insulin early this morning, didn't you? I knew it. It doesn't matter that it's worked out before. It didn't this time, did it? There must be more. I'll only go harder on you if you don't confess. You do feel guilty, don't you? You wouldn't feel that way if you hadn't done something wrong. You're hopeless and you know it."

It takes practice to turn down the volume on your Pushy Prosecutor so you can hear your Sympathetic Scientist, but you'll do yourself a great favor if you do just that.

June and Barbara: We've noticed that some people's Pushy Prosecutor is more interested in indicting them for high blood sugars than low blood sugars, even though lows are really more of a problem for these particular people because they often topple over the low borderline into reactions. Since the goal is a normal blood sugar, why do these people criticize themselves for being on the high side and think it's rather dandy to be low? Do they think it shows more strength of character if they avoid highs, whereas low blood sugars indicate that they've been working really hard on their diabetes—just maybe a little too hard?

Dr. Rubin: Yes, I think some people feel more guilty about highs than lows because they see highs as a sign of weakness and lows as a sign of virtue. These people may be into a too-much-of-a-good-thing syndrome. My son suffers from a variation on this theme. He's very proud of the fact that when he pushes the button on his meter that displays his average blood sugar value over the past several weeks, he usually gets a number like 113. Pretty impressive, isn't it? But the numbers that contribute to that average include many values over 200. He maintains his admirable record by having lots of lows. He takes clear pleasure in adding a low (like a 36!) to his meter database, as reflected by comments like, "That pulled my average down almost a whole point!"

This too-much-of-a-good-thing syndrome reminds me of people, diabetic and nondiabetic alike, who carry dieting or exercise to an extreme. They have trouble accepting that anything pushed to the limit can be destructive.

June and Barbara: Do you think the fear of getting complications from high blood sugar may have something to do with their wanting to push their lows to the limit?

Dr. Rubin: Definitely. Everyone knows about the risk of complications from chronic high sugars, so they feel guilty when they run high. Most believe there is no long-term risk from having lots of low reactions. Unfortunately, this isn't true. First off, people can die from severe reactions. It doesn't happen often, but it does happen. Second, there's some evidence that having large numbers of low blood sugars may permanently affect mental functioning. To put this in the bluntest terms, we could call these effects brain damage, and technically speaking this would be correct, but I want to be clear about what these studies actually show. They find that people who have lots of reactions score consistently lower on certain tests of mental functioning than people who have few reactions. But these differences are usually so small that their effects—if any—on day-to-day living are impossible to estimate.

Much more research needs to be done in this area before we can say with confidence what the real effects of frequent reactions are. This research will be done, because this is currently a hot area of investigation. In the meantime, we already know enough to be cautious when it comes to pushing for the lowest possible blood sugars. The massive, ten-year, nationwide Diabetes Control and Complications Trial is trying to assess the costs and benefits of tight blood-sugar control. The results of this study, which should start appearing within the next year or so, will also help us gauge the short-term and long-term risks of frequent reactions.

June and Barbara: A common burden of guilt comes from situations where diabetics have to impose certain of their regimen requirements on family and friends. They may feel guilty about the dietary adjustments the family makes even though the changes will vastly improve the whole family's health and longevity. Some diabetics handle diabetes-imposed family life changes with relative ease, but others feel guilty and are uncomfortable when others have to make adjustments for them. How can one avoid both excessive egocentricity and excessive self-effacement? Is there a happy medium?

Dr. Rubin: I often hear from diabetics how bad it feels to have their diabetes affect their families and friends. Some feel guilty about diabetes-related emotional outbursts. One woman told me that one night she broke everything in her kitchen; her greatest worry, she added, was keeping her husband from divorcing her.

Other diabetics feel guilty because they perceive themselves as a burden to their families rather than a help. One of my patients went to stay with her daughter to help care for a newborn granddaughter. Her blood sugars went out of control and she ended up needing more care than she was able to provide.

A related source of guilt is feeling that you're not meeting your responsibilities to your family. A woman whose blood sugars were really high fell asleep and forgot to unlock the door for her two young children. They sat on the steps outside for hours, unable to rouse her. A man felt horrible because he could not baby-sit his own young daughter, who was petrified to be left alone with him after he had a serious insulin reaction while taking care of her. Sometimes this form of guilt can be so strong that it makes a person want to avoid relationships altogether. One young woman told me that she had just fallen in love, but that she couldn't dream of putting her boyfriend and a child they might have through life with diabetes.

How to deal with these guilty feelings? First, accept that anyone would feel bad about some of the situations I've described. It's hard enough to deal with the burden diabetes places on you personally; it can be much harder when people you love are affected. But getting bogged down in guilt only paralyzes you and keeps you from devoting your energy to making sure you have less to feel guilty about. Even worse, guilt isolates you and cuts you off from the people you love and need most.

People who love you can handle the disappointment and responsibility that come with the territory when you have diabetes. In fact, the love they feel for you makes them want to be helpful, supportive, and flexible. Trust that, and you can create a positive self-fulfilling prophecy. You'll have the confidence to take the best possible care of yourself. You'll be open, optimistic, and appreciative with your family and friends. Your diabetes will be a fact of life together, not a fact that dominates your life together.

For those of you who are struggling with guilt and having trouble shaking it, I advise you to get it out in the open. Talk to your family and friends about it. You may find that you're overestimating the imposition they feel. Whether or not that's true, ask them how they would like to handle situations that trigger your guilt. You might also try asking other diabetics what tricks they have found helpful for banishing the "guilties."

June and Barbara: Sometimes we talk to diabetics who aren't doing very well with their self-care and who feel guilty and put down by others who have good control and seem to be doing everything right. What advice can you give these people to help them work their way out of this odious-comparison kind of dilemma?

Dr. Rubin: Although this isn't a common problem, it's a serious one for some people. One young man said to me forlornly, "I see people who seem to be able to stick to their diets, test their blood four times a day, exercise like they're supposed to, and keep their blood sugars close to normal almost all the time. When I see that it can be done, it makes me feel even worse about myself, like I'm a complete failure."

When you talk to people who seem to be doing so much better with their diabetes and you start to get down on yourself, stop for a moment. Remember that guilt is a wasted emotion that disables you from doing what you want to do. Just cut to the chase. Are these other people doing something you choose to incorporate into your regime? If so, great. How could you do it? If you don't waste all that energy getting down on yourself, you'll probably have enough left to begin answering this question. And beginning is really all you need to do to get yourself going.

June and Barbara: What if you don't choose to do something someone else is doing? Does this mean you're stuck with your guilt?

Dr. Rubin: If you don't want to do something, fine. Why get bent out of shape about it? That just seems like another form of wasted energy. The fact that someone else is doing the "right" thing is not a good enough answer. The only good enough answer is that you choose to make the change. If this sounds like a nonsensical position, I must tell you that I've seen literally hundreds of diabetics try to motivate themselves by guilt, but I've never seen one succeed. That's why I keep telling you that guilt is a wasted emotion. If it worked, I might be able to support the discomfort it involves. But it doesn't work. To help you get started thinking of a way to incorporate any changes you choose, try talking with your Sympathetic Scientist.

June and Barbara: To what extent do you think people who develop complications blame themselves and feel guilty? Doesn't this simply add an additional burden of mental distress?

Dr. Rubin: Complications are the great bogeyman for all diabetics. When the bogeyman actually makes an appearance, people often look for someone or something to blame. Some diabetics do blame themselves. Most of them know that poor self-care usually leads to poor diabetes control and that people in poor control are more likely to develop complications. As one man said to me, "I've had diabetes for 17 years and never had the willpower to take care of it. Now I'm paying the price. I had a stroke last month."

I've noticed, however, that often the blame for complications is laid on someone else's doorstep. Diabetics who were diagnosed when they were very young often see parents as the culprits. Parents who did not stress tight control are popular targets for this kind of retroactive guilt-tripping. The same criticism is often applied to doctors who condoned or even advocated loose self-care practices. I once treated a 34-year-old man who was preparing for penile implant surgery to deal with his impotence. He raged at the doctors who had treated him while he was growing up, and at his parents for allowing him to get away with poor control. He had depended upon them and they failed him, leading to his present agonized state. In his rage, this man forgot that there was a time when many doctors believed that tight control was impossible to achieve safely and was of no clear benefit, anyway. These were the days before home blood-glucose monitoring and before we had strong evidence about the benefits of tight control for delaying or preventing complications.

Other diabetics blame present-day family members for contributing to their poor control. They claim their family gives them no support and causes them emotional stress.

June and Barbara: We're surprised that so much of the blame is put on others rather than on the lack of good therapies or on self-neglect. Is some kind of self-delusion at work here?

Dr. Rubin: I think that blaming others is usually an effort to escape a burden of responsibility that would otherwise fall squarely on the shoulders of the diabetic. The essence of the problem here is that indulging in blame, either of others or of yourself, merely causes you more mental distress. More important, it paralyzes or distracts you; it *dis*ables you at the precise moment when focused, constructive action is most important. To successfully meet the challenge of complications, you need to mobilize all your inner resources and all the support that others may offer. You need to *en*able yourself. There's still so much to cherish and enjoy in your life.

June and Barbara: Here's a situation that has happened to June more than once. The hostess at a dinner party announces with pride that she has made a special dessert just for June. "It has no sugar at all—only honey!" As we all know, honey is just as bad as sugar for a diabetic. What do you do? You feel guilty if you don't eat the dessert, since the hostess has gone to so much trouble. Yet if you eat it, you're going to run your blood sugar up, which will make you feel guilty or angry or both.

Sometimes June eats just a taste or two, explaining that since she has already eaten so much of the delicious dinner, she is only allowed a little bit of the wonderful dessert. But should you allow the hostess to labor under the delusion that honey is okay for diabetics? If it's a good friend you can be frank and explain the facts of concentrated sweets. (Although you'd do it later, not in the company of the other guests, since that would embarrass the hostess and probably bore the others.) If it's a casual acquaintance, how far do you go in diabetes education?

Insulin-taking diabetics have a slight advantage in this kind of awkward dining situation, since they can always go home and take a little insulin to get back to normal. Type II's are stuck unless they want to do something like take a four-mile walk (in the middle of the night) to bring their blood sugar down.

To sum up, how far do you need to go to avoid embarrassing a host or hostess and avoid creating guilt for yourself by eating to be polite and running up your blood sugar? Any tips on how to handle this in the way that is psychologically best for everyone concerned?

Dr. Rubin: I'd say that June's approach is perfect for dealing with the situation on the spot. One of my patients called this the "no-thank-you-piece" technique. You accept a piece so small that it almost amounts to saying no thank you. This generally works. It avoids hurting the feelings of your host or hostess, and it avoids a major sugar overload. As you mention, this technique works best if you're on insulin and can simply take an extra unit or two of Regular to cover what you've eaten. If you take pills or if you really don't want to add even a few calories to your diet, you might try a variation on June's approach. You might say that you're so full you couldn't do justice to the glorious dessert, but could you take a piece home? You know just when you'll eat it, and it would be such a treat. Whether or not you actually eat the dessert later is up to you.

If you want to enlighten your host or hostess about concentrated sweets for diabetics, you'll need to say something later. As you point out, this is pretty easy if you're dealing with a good friend. If it's a casual acquaintance, the approach should be the same, though you might have to go more gently. Be sure that you state clearly how delicious the dessert was and how much you appreciated the thoughtfulness. Then you have to get to the bottom line, which is hard to sugarcoat. You explain that all concentrated sweets, including honey, have a similar effect on blood sugar and that this is very confusing unless you're a well-educated diabetic yourself. That's why you had to restrict yourself to a little piece, which was hard to do since it was so delicious. You might add that even though it's hard to resist sweet treats, you've found a couple of "safe" desserts you like. Extend an invitation to share one of them.

That's about all you can do, and it should be enough. If someone gets huffy when you approach him or her as gently and appreciatively as this, you need feel no guilt. You've done everything you could to be constructive.

➤ Help for Those Who Want to Help Diabetics

June and Barbara: It frequently happens—take it from Barbara, *very* frequently—that a nondiabetic family member or friend gets irritated, bored, or outright angry when a diabetic stops the action to take care of some situation. You can be all ready to go out and the diabetic has to take a blood sugar. You can be all ready to sit down at the dinner table and it turns out that the diabetic has high blood sugar so you have to delay (and possibly ruin) the meal until it comes down. Or you're planning a meal (either at home or out) for 7:00 P.M. and it's 5:45 and the diabetic's blood sugar plummets so you have to come up with some food or start the meal early (if you can!) and thereby spoil the planned rhythm of the evening.

It begins to seem as if the world revolves around the diabetic's needs and desires and never around yours, and you resent it. After all, you're a person with needs and desires, too. Why do you always have to be the one to make adjustments?

You may not even give voice to these feelings—in fact, you probably won't—but they're gnawing at you and, when you stop to think about it, making you feel guilty. After all, diabetics can't help doing all these things that spoil the fun and louse up the schedule . . . or could they help it if they tried? Whoops, there goes more guilt. Here you are accusing a hapless diabetic of either deliberately ruining things or ruining them because of handling the disease poorly. How do you handle these negative feelings and the guilt that they engender?

Dr. Rubin: These feelings do come up, and they are tough to deal with. That's why I say that if you love, live with, or care for a diabetic, you are living with diabetes, too. It doesn't affect your life in the same way that it does your diabetic loved one's life, but it affects it just as surely. You feel disappointed, upset, even angry or resentful on the one hand, yet on the other hand you feel guilty for having these feelings.

How do you avoid stewing in silence or exploding in anger (which would make you feel even more guilty)? The points I made in the Anger chapter about passive, aggressive, and assertive approaches to negative feelings apply here. You need to be assertive to avoid sliding into passivity or rage.

June and Barbara: How would this work at one of those excruciating moments when you're feeling simultaneously put upon and guilty?

Dr. Rubin: There are two ways to handle this that generally work. First, you could say, "I'm disappointed" (or upset, or whatever word accurately reflects your feeling). "We don't need to talk about it now, but I'd like to when we have a chance." Then follow through when the time is right, whether it's a few minutes, a few hours, or a few days later.

Second, if the situation is fairly calm, you could try to do some problem-solving right on the spot, in hopes of getting some of your needs met. Let's say your loved one needs some food to deal with a low blood sugar, and a special dinner you've been dreaming about for the past six weeks is only 90 minutes away. You might see if a small snack would save the day for both of you.

Whatever you do on the spot, there's always the opportunity for being assertive later, at some warm, comfortable moment when you're both feeling relaxed. This approach is especially important if the difficulty you're facing seems chronic.

June and Barbara: Could you show us how to handle this in a way that doesn't upset you both and cause more problems than it solves?

Dr. Rubin: Start by simply identifying the problem as you see it and explain your interest in the situation. For example: "I feel that we often end up running late for things because testing and shots come right at the last moment. I realize I tend to be compulsive about getting places on time and I also realize that you need to do your test and take your shot just before we leave the house. It would be great if we could work out an approach that meets both of our needs. Let's put our heads together and see if, in a spirit of mutual love and cooperation, we can come up with something."

This kind of loving assertion is important at many different levels. First, you feel better, not bottled up or raging. Second, you get some of your needs addressed. Third, your diabetic partner ends up feeling less like a burden. That's good for you, good for your partner, and good for your relationship.

June and Barbara: And good for cleaning out your guilt glands!

CHAPTER 9

EMBARRASSMENT
AN EMBARRASSMENT
OF EMBARRASSMENTS

Mark Twain said, "Man is the only animal that blushes. Or needs to." When it comes to blushing, literal or figurative, diabetics seem to do more than their share. They are embarrassed to be seen performing their therapies or eating their necessary snacks or glucose tablets, and they cringe at the thought of creating a scene by asking for special treatment in public situations like dining in a restaurant or flying on an airline and in more private situations like going out on a date or having dinner at a friend's house or traveling with a friend or in a tour group.

The sad part is that much of this embarrassment is only in the mind of the embarrassed one. The truth about people is that most of us are so self-absorbed and worried about embarrassing ourselves that we hardly notice situations that are bringing acute embarrassment to someone else.

It's also true that the older you grow the less frequently you experience the excruciating embarrassment of youth. Chronic embarrassment is one of the features that make being a teenager such agony and being a diabetic teenager pure hell. You could think of embarrassment as a kind of growing pain that you develop immunity to later in life. Maybe getting rid of embarrassment is one of the greatest comforts and compensations of age.

Embarrassment may seem like a small-potatoes negative emotion when compared to more significant ones like denial, grief, and fear. But embarrassment looms large on the diabetic emotional landscape if it causes you to neglect the diabetes therapies that insure your health and longevity.

Several years ago, a Cancer Society public-service ad appeared in women's magazines with the headline, "Aunt Edith Died of Embarrassment." The gist of it was that Aunt Edith was too embarrassed to go to the doctor for a Pap smear or breast examination. We don't want you to follow in Aunt Edith's footsteps. We don't want you to develop complications that could lead to disability and premature death out of embarrassment, so we'll ask Dr. Rubin to help you wipe that blush off your face and replace it with an expression of poise and confidence.

—June and Barbara

June and Barbara: People are often mortally embarrassed by very small things—for example, eating a necessary glucose tablet or a snack.

Dr. Rubin: That's true. One of my patients reported the following incident: "I was at my boyfriend's parents' 25th wedding anniversary and during dinner I felt an insulin reaction coming on so I had to go get my glucose pills. All the people at the table asked me what they were. When I told them that I had diabetes, they treated me like a baby and it seemed like they felt sorry for me. I hated it."

June and Barbara: If taking a glucose tablet embarrassed her that much, it would seem that a little judicious deception would be in order. She could pretend she needed a Kleenex or to make a phone call or to go to the bathroom (although that might have embarrassed her, too). Whatever the excuse, she could have taken her glucose in private and no one would have been the wiser.

Fortunately, in most situations you can subtly slip a glucose tablet or Lifesaver into your mouth without anyone even noticing. When it comes to taking a needed snack, you can become a popular favorite by carrying enough to be able to share your snacks with others—although that could run into money if you did it your whole life long. Fortunately, after a while people you know will have seen you snacking so often that you'll no longer be so embarrassed that you feel you have to feed everyone in sight when you need to eat.

Embarrassment at taking glucose tablets or eating snacks will probably quickly fade when we consider the alternative: having a major insulin reaction. For most Type I people, that can be the most embarrassing happening in their lives. We must admit that reaction behavior can be extremely bizarre. One man, Joe Brink, a muscle-builder who was Mr. Cincinnati in 1973, confessed to us that once in the hospital the nurses found him sitting nude on the over-the-bed table quacking like a duck while in the throes of a reaction. He was lucky to have this happen in the hospital, where the nurses and staff understand such goings-on. How do you overcome your feelings of chagrin when you do something weird in a less clinical environment?

Dr. Rubin: These things do happen. In fact, every Type I I know has had at least one really embarrassing reaction. Sometimes, as you mention, reactions have a bizarre, humorous side. One woman told me that she woke up in the middle of the night with a very low blood sugar, staggered down to the kitchen, opened the oven door, sat down on it, and urinated.

It is social and work situations that cause people the worst embarrassment. In the chapter on fear we've already covered the main strategy for handling this: try to minimize your reactions without compromising your control, and always use a reaction as a learning experience to see if you can come up with some ideas for protecting yourself in the future.

When a reaction does happen and you are left feeling extremely embarrassed about how other people saw you, keep in mind that in most cases the attention focused on you is an expression of caring and concern, not of disrespect or pity, as many people tend to interpret it. It's how *you* think about it that really counts in how much distress it causes (or doesn't cause) you.

One of my favorite techniques for deflating these negative feelings is, of course, to play up the humorous aspect of any situation. Since many reactions have a humorous side, or at least some humorous potential, humor can be your best ally. For example, one woman told me the following story.

She and her husband were in Baltimore for a diabetes education program at Johns Hopkins. Her special problem was reactions in the middle of the night. They were scary and often led to protracted arguments with her husband, since both were unnerved by the experience.

While they were in Baltimore, they were staying with their son and his family. Sure enough, one night she had a capital R Reaction. The situation was even worse than at home, because they ended up in the kitchen at 3 A.M. with their son, daughter-in-law, two grandchildren, and several household pets. When they got some cola and juice down her and the worst was over and everyone else had been shooed off to bed, the couple sat at the kitchen table with a dark cloud of embarrassment and discomfort over their heads.

Suddenly the woman remembered something I had said the day before about using humor to relieve bad feelings. Since she had to eat something more to get through the rest of the night, she made a couple of little peanut butter sandwiches. Then, spreading her robe on the floor, she sat down and patted a place inviting her husband to join her. "Here," she said, handing him a sandwich, "isn't this a perfect time and place for a picnic? There aren't even any ants!"

That did the trick. They both laughed, enjoyed their sandwiches, and felt fine again.

June and Barbara: That, of course, was a reaction *en famille*. Can humor be as effective in public with people you don't know that well?

Dr. Rubin: Humor can work almost anywhere. It helps relieve everyone's tension. My favorite example of using humor to turn around an embarrassing situation was a true story told to me by a friend. It didn't deal with diabetes, but it happened in public and it was certainly embarrassing enough for most purposes.

Two families who lived in Washington, D.C., were very good friends. Then one of the families moved to Alaska, and for years all communication was by letter and phone. Finally a reunion in Washington was arranged. As a highlight of the visit, both families went to a very fancy restaurant.

To start the evening off right, they ordered the most expensive red wine on the menu. The wine steward did his thing with the bottle and poured a sip for the oldest member from the Alaskan family to taste. The man held his glass aloft, looked at the color, sniffed the bouquet, took a sip—and choked! The wine came gushing out of his nose, all over the pristine white tablecloth. Without missing a beat, the man looked up at the wine steward, smiled, and said, "That's how we do it in Alaska."

Obviously this man was quick on his feet, but humor is more of a skill than a talent, so his wit is something to which we can all aspire. Someone once said to me, "Have you noticed that sooner or later we look back on everything and laugh, no matter how difficult the experience might have been at the time? So why wait? Laugh now!"

June and Barbara: A certain percentage of Type I diabetics are embarrassed to take insulin injections in public, while others do this all the time and think nothing of it. Why are attitudes so different on this issue and whose is healthier psychologically? Some people are even hesitant to test their blood sugar in public places, especially since the AIDS epidemic and the new feeling about the dangers of blood.

Dr. Rubin: Unfortunately, feeling embarrassed about taking shots in public is sometimes a well founded discomfort. I had a patient who took insulin in a public bathroom in a Miami airport and was reported to the police, who handcuffed him, frisked him, demanded to see his prescription for insulin (which he did not have with him), and held him past the time his plane took off before releasing him.

I had another patient, a 10-year-old girl whose father gave her her shot in the parking lot of a McDonald's before they went in to dinner. Apparently, someone reported this to the security guard of the restaurant, and when they entered, the father was aggressively confronted on the subject of giving his daughter drugs.

June and Barbara: June once became the focus of attention on a Paris street. She was sitting on a bus stop bench taking her insulin before entering a restaurant that she knew had a single small, dark unisex bathroom she wanted to avoid. She was so absorbed in what she was doing that until she looked up, she didn't realize she was creating something of a street scene. Parisians were staring so hard at her bizarre activity that a couple of them, walking backwards to be able to keep watching, crashed into lampposts. On the other hand, she has never been a focus of attention when taking a blood sugar, even though she does it anywhere and everywhere, including in the lobby during intermission at the theater and concerts. Probably people just think she's working out with her calculator or, when it makes sounds, her beeper.

Dr. Rubin: Blood tests don't usually draw as intense responses as taking insulin, although curious stares can sometimes be unwelcome. It's true, though, that seeing a diabetic take a blood-sugar test makes some people squeamish. I heard last week from the mother of a 7-year-old patient who had been testing her child's blood in an out-of-the-way spot at a relative's house. When the relative came upon them, she told them in no uncertain terms that she wanted all medical procedures conducted in the bathroom.

Of course, aside from a few extreme cases, most of the time people don't notice or don't care when you take your insulin or test in public. I think diabetics differ so much about whether they feel okay doing this because they differ so much in their need for privacy in all areas of life. I see the choice of how open you are about your shots as a purely personal matter, with no connotations of psychological health or lack thereof attached to either choice, as long as your choice doesn't compromise your care. Whether you take your shot at home before you go out, in your car, in a public restroom, or at a restaurant table is nobody's business but yours. But if your need for privacy leads you to skip shots or take them too early or too late, it's not okay. If this is your tendency, you need to consult your Sympathetic Scientist to see if you can come up with ways to protect your privacy without compromising your control.

You might decide that you don't need to be as private as you thought you did. This was the experience of one of my patients, Diana, a woman who never did her blood-sugar tests or took her insulin in front of her parents. In fact, although they certainly knew she had diabetes, she never even allowed herself to talk to her parents about her disease and her therapies. As a result she felt very isolated from them. Recently her parents took her out to a restaurant to celebrate her birthday. To protect her privacy (yes, from her own parents!), she had taken her shot before she left her house to meet them. When dessert time arrived she decided on the spur of the moment that she really wanted a treat, but she hadn't taken enough insulin to accommodate extra carbohydrate. There she sat trying to decide what to do. Should she skip the dessert and feel deprived? Should she eat the dessert and risk a very high blood sugar by waiting until she got home to take extra insulin? Should she quietly excuse herself to go to the bathroom without telling the truth? "No!" she thought, "This is my chance to break my silence."

She got up and said, "I'm going to go shoot up so I can have some of that delicious dessert." She obviously had a nice sense of humor to put it that way. She was feeling nervous, fearful of her parents' reaction when she returned to the table. Thoughts raced through her mind. "The worst I can imagine is that they won't say a word." Then she corrected herself. "No, the worst is that they won't be there when I get back, and they will have left me with the bill." As it turned out, Diana had nothing to fear. Her parents had been waiting for her to finally open up about her diabetes, so they were as happy to talk as she was. The next time she may even feel comfortable enough with them—and with her diabetes—to take the shot right at the table.

June and Barbara: Maybe it will help people like Diana be more open and less embarrassed about handling their diabetic procedures in public if they adopt the Dave Groves attitude. Dave, a veteran of 36 years of diabetes, is the head of the CompuServe Diabetes Forum (which we'll be discussing later). Dave reasons that everybody else in a restaurant is testing their blood sugars and administering their insulin every minute. You just can't see them doing it because it's automatically taking place inside their bodies. So why shouldn't you be able to do the same—even if it means pulling out your shirt or blouse and sticking yourself in the tummy at the table? "The restroom is the least sterile place in the restaurant," Dave maintains. "Why would you want to go there for your test and injection?"

Of course, people wearing an insulin infusion pump have little or no problem with taking their insulin in public since they're taking their basal (body maintenance) dose constantly, just as all the civilians in the room are. When they bolus (take an extra measure of insulin before eating), a casual observer would just think they're checking their beeper or tuning a very small radio.

Dr. Rubin: Even pumpers can have their moments of minor embarrassment. My friend and colleague, Cindy Miller, nurse-educator at the Johns Hopkins Diabetes Center, told me a couple of stories she heard at a meeting of her Insulin Pump Club. One of the pumpers said his pump came off his belt at one point and a friend commented, "Your pancreas is swinging." Another pumper was on a date once and pulled out her pump to bolus. Her date quickly interjected, "Oh no, I'm paying." She laughed and explained what she was doing. Almost always, a sense of humor turneth away embarrassment.

June and Barbara: Since most social events involve food and drink, many diabetics feel uncomfortable because they can't participate fully. For instance, they can't eat a slice of the wedding cake or they have to refuse all of the special sweets the hostess prepared for the occasion. It's also awkward to watch others eat and praise food while you stand by. Sometimes you even feel that you're making other guests uncomfortable because in their view you're deprived and they feel bad that you can't have what they're having. How can you put them and yourself at ease in these circumstances?

Dr. Rubin: You might feel like lecturing them on the evils of sugar, fat, and alcohol and quoting scientific evidence on the serious health risks inherent in consuming these substances. You might even feel like pointing out that by abstaining you may well live a longer and healthier life than they. You might *feel* like doing that, but, of course, that would really make them uncomfortable and you might not ever get invited again.

You have to be sensitive to other people's feelings, though they may not always be to yours. One woman told me that she hated to go out to dinner with friends. She knew what she should eat, but invariably one of them would announce to the waiter, in tones loud enough for everyone in the room to hear, that she had ordered what she had because she had diabetes. Understandably, this lady felt like sinking under the table. I advised her that if she did sink under the table, she might make herself useful down there by taking a bite out of the leg of the person who had made the comment.

Most people are much less obvious about their concerns for the diabetic's diet. How you deal with these situations depends on your goals. If you want to put other people at ease so you can relax yourself, you might try a script that goes something like this: "It's true that I miss certain goodies at times, especially as delectable-looking ones as those spread before me at the moment. But I've learned to get lots of pleasure out of just a little taste of these special treats [assuming you're going to let yourself have a taste]. Besides, I've also learned to enjoy vicariously foods I can't have myself. So I'm happy seeing you enjoy yourselves. I'd love to hear how that pie tastes, for instance."

This approach is likely to put others at ease, if you can pull it off. You don't have to really mean it completely; you just have to mean it enough to say it with a reasonable degree of conviction. If you can manage that, you may even convince yourself that it's true.

June and Barbara: Funny thing, but that's more or less the method June worked out for herself years ago (so it must be right!). But she carries it to the extreme in her thoughts. She actually feels sorry for people as she watches them eat too much and the wrong things, and we're afraid she wouldn't be up to telling them she was happy watching them enjoy themselves with unhealthy food. But that's just *her* way.

Now we come to another social hazard of somewhat an opposite nature. How can you keep people from fussing over you and cooking special food just for you? Men, especially, react negatively to being singled out this way or putting others to extra trouble.

Dr. Rubin: People differ in this respect. Some love to be catered to, others abhor it. If you're in the latter group, you hate to have people fuss over you. Unfortunately, there's no surefire way to get other people to stop doing this sort of thing or to make yourself comfortable with it. The best I can do is offer a few suggestions that may help a bit.

First, try to keep in mind that this kind of attention is an indication of caring and love. If part of your discomfort is a fear that people are fussing for any other reason, this realization ought to ease your mind to some extent.

Second, you can have a chat in private with the fusser and explain, without hurting his or her feelings, that you really appreciate the thoughtfulness, but you're kind of shy and prefer not being singled out. Even though you recognize the person's good intention, you can't help having this odd quirk in your nature. Explain that it's not necessary to prepare anything special for you. You can have a *little* of almost anything, and that's the arrangement that suits you best.

The main thing to remember is that in this delicate situation, tender treatment of the other person is what's called for.

➤ Help for Those Who Want to Help Diabetics

June and Barbara: Diabetics often don't want to call attention to themselves by requesting special treatment—no matter how necessary that special treatment may be. Barbara solved this one by pretending to be the diabetic and asking for these things as if they were for her. Since she isn't a diabetic, it doesn't embarrass her in the slightest to ask for virtually anything.

For example, when we want to check out a menu at a restaurant to see if it's appropriate before deciding whether to eat there, Barbara marches up to the person at the desk and announces, "I have diabetes and I need to look over your menu to see if I can find some dishes that are on my diet." Then the two of us proceed to pore over the menu.

You could say that you don't even have to mention diabetes, just ask to see the menu. That's true. But if it turns out there's nothing that fits into the diabetic diet—or more likely nothing you want that fits into the diabetic diet—it's less offensive to say, "I'm sorry, I can't find something that's on my diet" than it is to just hand back the menu and leave. (Restaurateurs have feelings, too!)

Barbara also sometimes claims to be the diabetic when June's blood sugar is going down and she needs to be seated and served right away. The one thing wrong with this scheme is that sometimes the waiter or waitress will keep hovering around Barbara making sure that everything's all right and that there's nothing else she needs.

Her greatest coup in this regard occurred several years ago at De Gaulle airport in Paris. They announced that our flight was delayed three hours. We had selected that flight because it served lunch and it was time for lunch. Two hours later would throw June off schedule.

Barbara went to the airline desk and asked if they were planning to serve the passengers meals at the airport as they often do in the case of long delays. No, they hadn't planned to do that. They would serve lunch after the plane took off in three hours. Barbara started protesting vehemently that this would do her no good because she was a *diabétique* and she had to eat right now or (ominously) there would be Big Trouble.

The desk attendant's hand was quicker than the eye as she opened a drawer and pulled out two meal vouchers—the only two she distributed that day—for the best airport restaurant. There we enjoyed a delicious three-course French meal (including wine) that was far better, far more appropriate for a diabetic, and far more on time than the airline meal would have been. In fact, we enjoyed ourselves so much that we lost track of time and almost missed the plane when it finally did take off.

If it had been up to June to protest, she probably would have just knuckled under and eaten a soggy sandwich from the nearby snack stand. But, as we said, that was several years ago and the intervening years have diminished June's embarrassment and increased her assertiveness. She now asks for most of her diabetic needs herself, figuring she could do it more gracefully and effectively than the *diabétique imaginaire.*

The diabetic in your life likewise may appreciate having someone else take the flak in the early days when embarrassment is in full bloom, but later on will probably prefer to handle situations himself or herself.

Another helpful thing you can do is to run interference for the diabetic when it comes to dining at friends' houses. Many times hosts or hostesses ask Barbara ahead of time (with an air of desperation), "What can June eat, anyway?" It's then easy to set their minds at ease with a quick rundown of what's okay. This is a good opportunity to solve that eternal "I-made-the-dessert-especially-for-you-it-has-no-sugar-at-all-only-honey" problem.

Even if they don't ask, it's easy to anticipate the situation by saying something like, "You may have been wondering about what Edgar can eat because of his diabetes. I want to assure you that he can eat almost anything everyone else does as long as he knows what's in it and as long as it doesn't contain concentrated sweets like sugar, honey, molasses, and such." At this time, you can also find out approximately when dinner will be served so Edgar can plan his injection (assuming that Edgar is on insulin).

It just takes a little preliminary groundwork for you to diminish the potential for embarrassment on both sides of the dinner table, and everyone will be happy you did it—including you.

Dr. Rubin, do you have any other tricks of the trade that you and the family members of your patients have come up with to ward off diabetic embarrassment?

Dr. Rubin: Barbara and June, I take my hat off to you. It's hard to think of anything I've tried or even heard of that you haven't covered. The only thing I can add is a general suggestion for people who haven't yet developed the wonderful cooperation you've achieved. If you're a person just getting started trying to emulate some of the ways Barbara takes the pressure off June, make sure you're pursuing your diabetic loved one's agenda and not your own.

CHAPTER 10

PSYCHOLOGICAL HELP
SHRINKING YOUR PROBLEMS

In the lexicon of light-bulb jokes, one of our favorites is: "How many psychotherapists does it take to change a light bulb? Answer: Only one, but it can take a very long time and the light bulb has to really want to change."

As with many jokes, this one contains a lot of truth. Most of us human light bulbs, even though we may be sitting there burnt out and in the dark, don't *really* want to change. Change is hard. Change is disruptive. Change is risk-taking. Change is scary. We resist change with every fiber in our being. Oh, we may declare, "I'm going to shape up," or "Don't worry, I'll get my act together," but deep down inside there's that loud voice shouting "NO!"

But diabetes has an equally loud voice shouting, "*Change.* That's what I'm all about. Get yourself right with me, or you're in for Big Trouble." You don't know how to come to terms with these conflicting messages. Your diabetes keeps demanding change; your inner self keeps saying no.

It takes a lot of strength and courage to fight your change-resisting enemy within. You need allies in the battle. Friends and family members try to help, and sometimes succeed, but if the enemy within is particularly strong and powerful—as it often is—you need to enlist help from professional warriors of the psyche who have studied tactics and have helped others fight and win their battles for change.

Often all those around you can see that you need this help—even you can see you're not making it by yourself—but here comes that loud inner voice again shouting, "NO! I'm not weak. I'm not crazy. I don't need a shrink. I can handle this thing myself. Leave me alone."

If you find yourself in this double-negative state, we're now going to ask Dr. Rubin to eliminate the negative. Cardinal Newman said, "To live is to change." Dr. Rubin will show you how to say YES! to help, YES! to change, and YES! to life.

—June and Barbara

June and Barbara: The first rather obvious question is how do you know if you need professional help? Can you tell us the most common kinds of emotional problems people enter psychotherapy to solve, to give us an idea of who needs such help and who doesn't?

Dr. Rubin: There are two main reasons to seek professional help. First, if you have a major psychological disorder such as depression, anxiety disorder, obsessive-compulsive disorder, or an eating disorder, it is essential to get professional help, because you're taking an unnecessary risk with your physical health if you don't. Every one of these conditions severely hampers your ability to take good care of your diabetes.

Second, people often seek counseling when they feel bogged down and unable to cope with the demands of daily life with their disease. People in this category are not really psychologically disturbed in a clinical sense. They're just burned out or overwhelmed. If this is your problem, you need some solid support from a professional who knows how to help psychologically intact but emotionally exhausted people get back on the right track.

June and Barbara: We once heard a radio psychologist say that if you won't make changes in your life, you aren't miserable enough. Do you think that misery breeds change? Do certain people have to be hit over the head with something as misery-inducing as the beginnings of complications before they're willing to shape up?

Dr. Rubin: The psychologist you quote is expressing the common notion that you have to hit bottom before you can locate your motivation for change. Unfortunately, this is often true. I mentioned in the Denial chapter that many people are not motivated to do the right thing by the prospect of complications. Only the reality seems to move them.

I'm an optimist, though. In fact, we've based this book on the hope, even the expectation, that with the proper tools, people can locate their motivation for positive change without having to hit bottom. People stop denying when the costs of this approach get so heavy that they outweigh its benefits. That's why complications often lead to positive change. But there's also another approach to locating the motivation you need to do the right thing: reducing the costs involved in doing it. The techniques we've talked about throughout this book are designed to do just that: to help you see that it's easier than you thought to deal directly with your diabetes. Reducing the costs of doing the right thing tips the balance just as surely as increasing the costs of denial, and it has the overwhelming advantage of setting your feet on the paths of diabetic righteousness *before* dire consequences befall you.

June and Barbara: Do most of your patients decide they need help and come in on their own or are they referred to you by M.D.s? We ask this because we remember you sent us a note you got from a patient who had asked his doctor for a letter prescribing counseling so that he could get insurance reimbursement for your services. The note from the M.D. read: "I do not refer patients to psychologists for diabetes mellitus. I do not know what their role would be."

Dr. Rubin: My referrals come from a variety of sources, including endocrinologists and other diabetes specialists, people I've seen in clinics at hospitals where I work, people who attend my lectures, and people referred by other patients.

The note you mention is one I'll never forget. It's sobering to think that there are doctors out there who treat lots of diabetics and are still unaware of the role emotions play in overall management. Treating any chronic disease as a strictly medical phenomenon misses much of what's really going on. Even though this doctor is not alone in his narrow view, I'm encouraged by the fact that more and more health-care professionals see things as they really are.

If your doctor is unaware of the role of emotions in diabetes, you would be doing yourself a great favor to try to educate the doctor. This might not be easy, but you don't want your doctor missing the boat when your health and well-being are at stake.

June and Barbara: By whatever route a diabetic reaches the therapist's door, what kind of therapies—and therapists—are likely to work best for them?

Dr. Rubin: It's safe to say that just about every form of therapy ever practiced has been tried at least once in the treatment of diabetes. I'm convinced that any approach can be helpful. The key is really the skills of the therapist, not his or her orientation. Besides, I've been in the therapy business long enough to have learned that good therapists tend to be more similar in their approach to patients than their nominal attachment to particular schools of therapy might suggest.

June and Barbara: If it's not so much the therapy as the therapist that matters, how do you know if you have the right one, the one who will be the most effective at helping you over the emotional hurdles?

Dr. Rubin: The number one consideration is that you need to feel comfortable with your therapist. I don't mean comfortable the way you do with a friend. I mean comfortable to say what's on your mind, comfortable that the therapist is listening carefully to what you say, comfortable that the therapist's comments to you reflect some basic understanding of what makes you tick and can lead you to stretch your own capacity to understand yourself.

Another crucial requirement is that the therapist have some basic understanding of diabetes. Psychological and emotional problems are often inextricably interwoven with a person's day-to-day life with diabetes. I couldn't treat people who have diabetes nearly as effectively if I didn't know how the disease affects their lives. Unfortunately, very few therapists specialize in treating people who have diabetes. A good test of whether a therapist is right for you might be his or her willingness to read the sections of this book you feel are most relevant to your situation—and, for background, to read a basic book or two on the physiology of diabetes and diabetes therapy.

June and Barbara: We'd like you to take us behind the closed door and tell us what you actually do in a counseling session, so that people will have some idea of what they're getting into if they're thinking about going to a therapist and thus will feel less apprehensive when they decide to give it a try. We don't expect you to give away any trade secrets (if they are secret), but most diabetics have never experienced psychotherapy and would appreciate a little preview.

Dr. Rubin: I could write a book about the basic counseling techniques I use. Come to think of it, we have! Actually, I've described my techniques in individual situations in every one of the previous chapters, so I'll just pull together an overview here.

I do two different kinds of counseling with diabetic patients. I provide training in diabetes-specific coping skills for those who have garden-variety diabetes-related problems in living. And I do what is called cognitive-behavioral psychotherapy with those who have diagnosable psychological disorders. The techniques for either group are based on the same approach: breaking the cycle of negative thought leading to negative feeling leading to negative behavior. Working your way out of this self-defeating pattern involves three steps:

1. Recognizing the power of basic beliefs and automatic thoughts to trigger cycles of emotion and action (or inaction).

2. Learning to tune into and identify your own unique system of beliefs and thoughts.

3. Practicing basic reframing techniques (shifting from a negative perception to a positive one) to create a mood where something good can happen. This lets you reach a place where you can achieve physical and emotional well-being.

Suggestions for the first two steps of this process appear throughout the previous nine chapters of this book. (You might go back to the Guilt chapter to see how this process worked with the woman who tended to snack all evening.) Suggestions for the third step are the subject of the next chapter.

June and Barbara: Since therapy is such an individual thing, we're certain that there must be a lot of variation within these two kinds of counseling. You probably wouldn't try to fit everyone into the same treatment any more than you'd try to fit them into the same pair of shoes.

Dr. Rubin: You're right. There are infinite variations but there are some basic patterns. In preparing to write this book, I looked over the files of the many people with diabetes who've come to me for private counseling. They came to me for a variety of reasons, and the best therapy for each one depended upon those reasons. Some people seem very well put together emotionally. They consult me because they're having a specific problem coping with some aspect of their lives with diabetes. My work with them is usually focused and brief. The process is active, with a lot of give-and-take, and our orientation is very much that of partners in problem solving. I talk a lot, offering guidelines, examples, encouragement, suggesting experiments, and the like.

A second group of people are suffering more deeply. They may be clinically depressed or anxious or they may suffer from obsessive-compulsive disorder. At the same time, these people seem to be functioning fairly well in general. They have reasonable relationships and do okay in school or work. Their emotional problems seem to be pretty clearly focused on diabetes. They probably had tendencies toward the same emotional difficulties before they developed diabetes, but these tendencies might have stayed under control forever if diabetes hadn't added to their burden. Work with these patients is slower and more involved, since the underlying psychological disorder has to be treated along with—sometimes even before—the diabetes coping issues.

In these cases I draw upon my experience as a general psychotherapist. When necessary, I recommend psychotropic medications prescribed by a psychiatrist with whom I consult. As the underlying psychological disorder resolves, which it does in most cases, we can complete the rest of the specifically diabetes-related work. Sometimes very little of this work remains, because for some people life with diabetes is a problem only when the disease is added to clinical psychological difficulties.

The third group of diabetics who consult with me have very serious psychological problems. Unfortunately, this is the largest group I see. This is not representative of the whole diabetic population. It's that the people who come to me are generally the most troubled.

June and Barbara: Now that you've given us such a clear picture of what kinds of patients you treat and how you go about treating them, we'd like to turn the tables and let a patient tell his side of the counseling story. At the opening of the Depression chapter we reprinted a letter from Alan, who was referred to a psychiatrist because of the extreme depression that the diagnosis of diabetes had caused him. To quote Alan, "Seeing a psychiatrist turned out to be the smartest thing I could have done." Here's Alan's story of his counseling experience exactly as he described it to us.

> The first thing the psychiatrist made clear to me was that what I was going through was neither uncommon nor particularly abnormal. She pointed out how I was going through the classic stages of grief (denial, anger, sadness, etc.) and emphasized that it was not only okay, but necessary to go through a period of adjustment. I had been hit with a serious blow and I needed time to deal with it. I also needed to separate out the diabetes-related issues from the non-diabetes-related issues affecting my depression. The process of therapy, I discovered, was really one of untangling the myriad of issues underlying my depression and then examining each one realistically with the guidance of a professional who has seen many people deal with similar situations and problems.
>
> Like diabetes, the more I learned about depression the less mysterious it became. Although it would be a few weeks before I learned to "manage" the depression much as one "manages" diabetes, I learned to be prepared for the mornings by forcing myself to do things that I knew I wouldn't want to do, but which I also knew I would be glad to have done. Things like exercising (especially swimming and bike riding) and getting a massage were consistently effective. Probably the hardest—and most important—task in managing my depression was to fight the overwhelming temptation to retreat into my own little depressed world. I was fortunate that I had both family and friends who never let me retreat completely. During one particularly bad spell, just after my diagnosis,

I had one brother who called practically every night and another who flew in from out of town. I also had a variety of friends who continued to call and invite me out, even though more often than not, I neither wanted to talk nor go out. Their persistence, aside from being just plain supportive, stopped me from completely isolating myself and ended up easing my transition out of depression.

Ironically, I first really sensed that the depression had lifted on a gambling trip to Atlantic City. The rush of winning gave a surge of pleasure that I hadn't experienced since my diagnosis. Gradually, as I spent more and more time doing things I always wanted to do but never seemed to have the time—things like painting, bike-riding, reading, and spending weekends at a Quaker retreat—it became increasingly clear that diabetes really did not stop me from enjoying life. As I returned to my work as filmmaker, it also became quickly evident that the diabetes in no way stopped me from pursuing my chosen career.

We think Alan's story shows realistically how therapists work with people to bring them out of the negative states that diabetes can induce. Alan was only in therapy a few months and at the conclusion he emerged cured. Is this a typical outcome? In other words, Dr. Rubin, what can you tell us about the success rate in diabetes counseling? Are any statistical measurements available?

Dr. Rubin: There are no statistical measurements available on the effectiveness of diabetes counseling. In an effort to correct this lack, I've started to create a database of my own patients and the results of their work with me. I've also launched an initiative to encourage other therapists who counsel substantial numbers of diabetics to do the same, so that we can pool our results. I hope it won't be long before I can offer a more reliable answer to your question.

June and Barbara: Do you ever have people come in for counseling whom you can't help, or, more likely, who drop out too early in the game?

Dr. Rubin: Yes, some people who come to me for counseling leave without much improvement or drop out before making much real progress. This is most often the case when people have very serious psychological problems. Their lives are in chaos and their diabetes is only one more, often relatively minor, source of distress. My work with these patients is often unsuccessful, especially when they come to me for only a few sessions. They're in such pain that they find little relief in our work.

Others stay with the work despite their pain. We work together for months, sometimes years. We struggle to resolve their nearly crippling difficulties with depression, anxiety, social isolation, or eating disorders. We take three steps forward and two backward. We count our victories on the smallest of scales and congratulate ourselves when we have any victories at all. Sometimes the small victories accumulate, and my patients' strides toward well-being lengthen. Sometimes, on the other hand, our work ends after years with only a handful of small successes. Whichever the case, I find that these long collaborations rarely end in disappointment. I'd like to think this is because we both know we did the best we could together. That's a rare and precious experience.

June and Barbara: Is there any way for a person to tell how long to stick with therapy? Just when should one reasonably start looking for improvement?

Dr. Rubin: Length of therapy is such an individual matter that it's hard to make general statements, but I'll try. If you've got the right therapy and the right therapist, you should begin to notice at least one thing pretty quickly: feeling a sense of trust and confidence in this person. You should feel that he or she really hears what you're saying and responds in a way that makes you comfortable.

Beyond that, the relevant issues are your goals and the nature of your problem. If your goals are primarily to improve your diabetes coping skills or to relieve the acute symptoms of depression or anxiety, you should expect some results within 10 to 12 sessions. That's not to say that your problems will be all gone within this time, but rather that you should get some meaningful relief by then. With certain symptoms of psychological distress, medication can dramatically cut the period of acute agony. If your goals are more in the realm of self-exploration, you should also get some important insights before too many weeks go by, though the changes may be less striking than with some of the other reasons for seeking therapy.

It's easy to say that you should realistically expect to see some fairly rapid improvement in the problem that brought you to therapy. It's harder to say how much total improvement you can expect over the entire course of treatment, or when it's time to stop. Feeling that you're basically okay or that a number of sessions have gone by without any discernible progress are two good reasons for raising the issue of stopping your therapy. I strongly suggest that you talk through your decision thoroughly with your therapist and think carefully about how he or she addresses your thoughts on the matter.

June and Barbara: We seem to keep talking here about people being reluctant to go into therapy or dropping out of it too soon. What if the opposite occurs? Maybe it's just because we're in California, but we've had friends who take to therapy too well. They almost become addicted to it. Although we can't know what personal demons they're wrestling with, they're successful in their careers and personal relationships and they seem as well-adjusted as the rest of us, but they keep going regularly to therapists—sometimes the same one and sometimes different ones—year after year. Is there a risk of becoming a therapy junkie?

Dr. Rubin: When you use the words *addicted* and *therapy junkie*, I assume you're talking about an unhealthy dependence.

I'm not sure how this would apply to involvement in therapy. On second thought, I can think of one way: if the therapy somehow kept a person from acting independently. There is some risk of this if the therapist and the patient lose sight of the primary goal of therapy—empowering the patient.

Sometimes this process of empowerment, helping the person become his or her own therapist, takes only a few weeks or months. Other times, when the person has serious psychological problems, the process can—just like changing the light bulb in the joke—take a very long time. But in either case, the goal is the same: fostering independence.

When I work with a person, I make this goal explicit and refer to it every session we meet, whether those sessions number two or two hundred. We're always oriented toward that conclusion. We can never be absolutely certain when the perfect moment has arrived to stop our work together. In fact, there probably is no such moment. So we make the wisest choice we can, clear about the fact that my door is always open. People sometimes come back for a brief tune-up, or even for a more extensive reengagement if they find they've stopped before they were truly ready or if some new problems arise. I find that this open-door policy makes it easier to stop the initial work sooner rather than later, and that's generally a plus.

Occasionally a patient wants to continue seeing me past the point where it seems therapeutically necessary from my point of view. I'll be candid when I think this is happening, and this generally leads to a constructive discussion of the patient's natural fears about operating without the support of therapy. This will usually move us toward concluding the therapy, though this last stage can take quite a while for certain people.

I guess I've wandered fairly far afield from your original question, so let me get back to it. While I do think it's possible for a person to become addicted to therapy, it's very unlikely if therapist and patient are both working to facilitate the person's ability to live independently.

June and Barbara: How can people go about finding a good, effective, and empowering therapist in their own community?

Dr. Rubin: This is a hard one. There are few central registries of therapists. Different mental-health professional groups—counselors, psychiatrists, psychiatric nurses, psychologists, social workers, and the like—tend to have their own registries. Here are some hints for finding a good therapist. If you feel that diabetes-related problems are part of the reason you're seeking counseling, you might try several sources: The American Association of Diabetes Educators (444 N. Michigan Ave., Suite 1240, Chicago, IL 60611-3901; phone 1-800-338-3633), which maintains a list of all Certified Diabetes Educators, including some who are mental-health professionals; your local American Diabetes Association affiliate; your diabetes doctor; a local hospital; someone you know who is seeing a good therapist; and people in your diabetes support group.

If you can't find a therapist who is knowledgeable about diabetes, at least find one who is willing to learn about it. If you think you might need medication for your emotional problems, look for a psychiatrist (a medical doctor able to prescribe drugs), or for a counselor who has a working relationship with a psychiatrist. If you're attracted by a particular psychotherapeutic orientation, such as the cognitive-behavioral approach I use, ask any counselor you see if he or she uses this approach. Try to get comfortable with the idea of interviewing prospective therapists. I know this is tough to do, especially when you don't know how you're supposed to feel with a therapist, but it's important to pay attention to the chemistry between the two of you. Fortunately, there are lots of good therapists, and if you're in need of help, it's important that you find one of them.

June and Barbara: Back in our college days there was a saying about joining fraternities and sororities: "35 friends at five dollars apiece." We've heard similar remarks about therapists—only the price is higher. You're buying yourself a very expensive friend, someone to discuss your problems with and support you during life's dark periods. When you come right down to it, what can a therapist do that an intelligent and sympathetic good friend can't?

Dr. Rubin: Therapy does cost quite a bit, so your question makes a lot of sense. I would definitely encourage anyone who's struggling emotionally to first try working out the problem with family and friends. Beyond that, a good therapist can do a lot that a friend can't. If you've tried unsuccessfully to solve your problems "at home," you probably already know most of what I'm going to tell you.

A therapist is disinterested, not uninterested. He or she is not involved in your problems in any way other than a profound professional concern for your well-being. He or she has no other stake in what you do or how you do it. This means that your therapist has no agenda of his or her own. A good therapist will not get frustrated and push you or get angry and walk away from you or get hurt and break down, as people who live with you and love you inevitably will. This disinterested attitude lets you do the work you need to do, the work only you can do, the work of figuring out what you're thinking and feeling and how to get things straight.

In addition, a good therapist has other professional skills that come with training and experience, skills that can be invaluable in helping you get unstuck. He or she can help you look past the obvious to see in new ways what's going on inside and around you. Based on these insights, your therapist can help you find new approaches to the problems that brought you to counseling. When we talk to our family and friends, we tend to tell variations on the same stories over and over again, and they tend to respond to us in ways that are similarly ritualized. We're often unaware of how predictably we communicate about our problems. A good therapist helps us get out of this rut, with potentially wonderful consequences.

June and Barbara: No matter how much we may want or need or would benefit from a professional therapist, most of us still have to be concerned with the cost. Just how much can we expect to pay for therapy?

Dr. Rubin: Fees range quite a bit, depending on the area of the country where you live and the professional credentials of the therapist. Psychiatrists tend to charge the highest fees, psychologists a bit less, and counselors, social workers, and psychiatric nurses a bit less than psychologists. I've heard of fees as high as $175 to $200 an hour and as low as about $40 an hour.

Many therapists charge on a sliding scale, which means that their fees are determined in part by the patient's ability to pay. Some therapists are "preferred providers" with certain insurance plans, which means that they have a contract with the plan to charge members a set (usually reduced) fee. When you first talk to a prospective therapist, make sure you get the facts on fees, sliding scales, and preferred provider arrangements, as well as the therapist's policy for payment. Some ask you to pay at each session or once a month and let you collect the insurance reimbursements. Others may agree to accept only your copayment and collect the rest directly from your insurance company. The latter arrangement can ease your cash flow.

June and Barbara: Speaking of reimbursements, do most private insurance plans and Medicare and Medicaid provide assistance in paying for psychological counseling?

Dr. Rubin: Health insurance plans of all sorts generally pay for counseling. In many states (my state of Maryland, for instance), mental-health benefits are mandated as part of all insurance plans. Medicare and Medicaid also reimburse. The amount of mental-health benefits varies by plan. Some reimburse as much as 80–90 percent of counseling fees; others as low as 40 percent. Some plans limit the number of sessions for which they will reimburse in a given year—typically 10, 20, or 50.

Some health maintenance organizations (HMOs) provide counseling at no cost or very low cost as part of their package of services. The downside is that they tend to limit allowable counseling services to crisis intervention for a very few sessions, and services must be provided by a therapist employed by the HMO. Because I offer a service (diabetes-specific counseling and coping skills training) rarely available with HMOs, patients who have these plans are sometimes able to obtain referrals from their HMOs to see me. Unfortunately, our work together must be very brief, since the plans will usually pay for no more than a handful of sessions.

June and Barbara: So far we've been discussing individual psychotherapy, but since diabetes is often called a family disease in the sense that the entire family lives with it and not just the diabetic, we're going to bring up the subject of family counseling. What's is it and in what kinds of family situations is it useful?

Dr. Rubin: Family therapy is an approach that includes all members of the family, even those who aren't obviously involved in the problem. Family therapists take this approach because they believe that everyone who lives with the problem *is* in some way involved in maintaining it and must therefore also be involved in solving it. In a sense, the family is the patient in family therapy. This approach can be especially useful when the diabetic family member is a child or adolescent, since it's so clear in these cases that other family members must be involved in solving the problem.

Family therapists identify, evaluate, and help correct patterns of family interaction and communication that don't work well. Families living with diabetes have been treated with this approach, especially families with diabetic children. Few of these efforts have been written up and published. I've had some success with family therapy myself. It makes a lot of sense to me. When I see diabetics, especially young people, whose control is terrible, I almost always find serious family problems as well. One endocrinologist once described the family lives of kids like these as "soap operas." It's tempting to say that the family problems have caused the control problems, and I'm sure there's a lot of truth in that. At the same time, the control problems may also be contributing to the family problems. What you have working is a very powerful negative cycle, which family therapy can help correct.

June and Barbara: We've had people tell us that they got a lot out of going to group therapy sessions that were run by various psychologists or hospitals. We've attended a few of these sessions and seen people actively participating and obviously benefiting from the interchange of ideas. Have you ever worked with group therapy?

Dr. Rubin: Yes, group therapy is an approach I've found useful. I've heard of therapy groups that brought together people with similar concerns—teenagers, parents of young diabetics, blind diabetics, for example. Other times membership of the group is less focused.

As with family therapy, there's little hard data on the effect of this approach, but some benefits have been identified, and they're consistent with the results of the groups I've run. Group therapy can help diabetics feel less isolated. It can also help people feel more comfortable with their diabetes and more willing to take good care of themselves in ways like increased openness about their disease, more frequent blood testing, and willingness to wear an identification bracelet. Because groups can help people take better care of themselves, they can also contribute to improved glycemic control.

Some groups are structured to train participants to deal effectively with diabetes-related situations like testing, shots, meals away from home, or stresses that contribute to slipping off the path of good self-care. I did a study of the outpatient education program at the Johns Hopkins Diabetes Center where I work, which includes a coping skills training component along the lines I just described. I found that when people graduated from the program, they had improved emotional well-being (higher self-esteem and lower depression and anxiety), improved self-care skills, and improved glycemic control. These improvements persisted 6 months and 12 months after the program ended. Some of the participants told me that the group coping skills training was essential to helping them feel better about themselves and to motivating them to put the education program into action.

You may have trouble finding a group like the ones I've described. If so, you may be able to get some of the same benefits from a good diabetes education program or a support group.

June and Barbara: Support groups were just what we were coming to. In the September/October 1991 issue of *Diabetes Educator,* Roberta J. Seevers reported that an estimated 15 million people in the United States belong to 500,000 support groups.

We once talked to a man from Minneapolis who claimed that his city was the greatest place for support groups in the world. He said that if you had an accident and lost the tip of the little finger on your left hand, you could instantly find a Minneapolis support group of others with lost left little fingertips to help you adjust to your loss.

These days even traditionally stoic and reticent men are joining support groups to discuss aspects of their masculinity. An article on the new men's movement in the June 24, 1991, issue of *Newsweek* quoted one participant in a weekend support group. He said that talking with other men that weekend he realized the importance of men learning from one another, because "alone we don't know what the hell we're doing."

Ms. Seevers' study indicated that currently there are more than 800 diabetes support groups in this country, apparently helping people learn "what the hell they're doing" about adjusting to diabetes. Do you think of these support groups as a form of therapy?

Dr. Rubin: Therapy is a pretty broad term. If we define it as professional help, support groups are not therapy. If, on the other hand, we define therapy as any structured approach to enhanced self-awareness and improved physical and emotional well-being, support groups can fill the bill. At their best, support groups probably provide many of the same benefits that therapy groups do. I say *probably,* because there's not a single study of the benefits of diabetes support groups.

Support groups do differ from therapy groups in a number of ways. Most prominently, support groups usually have no professional leader, and often no leader at all. They're usually open-ended. They're open to anyone and they go on for months or years, without a defined endpoint. Therapy groups are usually structured more formally and often operate for a set number of sessions. Support groups also tend to meet less often, perhaps once a month or so, while therapy groups usually meet weekly or every other week.

June and Barbara: What are some of the specific benefits of support groups?

Dr. Rubin: Like group therapy, the good ones probably help people feel less isolated, better about themselves, more comfortable with their diabetes, and more able to do the right thing when it comes to their self-care. In addition, support groups are free or, at most, require a small contribution. That's a real benefit. You're also more likely to be able to find a support group in your neighborhood than a diabetes therapy group. For these reasons, I always encourage people to join support groups. Not all groups are good ones, and even some good ones might not be right for you. But look for one you like, and keep looking until you find one. It can be a wonderful resource.

June and Barbara: Do you know of any risks involved in support groups?

Dr. Rubin: The only risk I can think of is that certain full-blown emotional problems are beyond a support group's ability to manage. Real depression, an anxiety disorder, or chronic self-destructive behavior probably won't be relieved without professional help. Even here, though, a support group can be helpful in encouraging the troubled person to seek therapy. As long as the group members don't try to manage problems they can't handle, I see no risks and lots of benefits to joining a support group.

June and Barbara: It's obvious from what you've said in answer to many of the questions on therapy that a major difficulty is finding help in your own community. Back when we started the SugarFree Center, we wanted to serve people in isolated places who had no access to new diabetes self-care information and products. We mentally created a mythical typical remote area where we felt our help was needed. We christened it West Buffalo Breath, Wyoming. When something new came along, we'd say to each other, we've got to let the folks out in West Buffalo Breath know about this!

Now there are plenty of mail-order services and diabetes publications, so the people in West Buffalo Breath are getting as sophisticated as the big-city folks about diabetes self-care. Still, they only have access to therapies for the body. It's not surprising that a small hamlet wouldn't have diabetes support groups, let alone therapists specializing in diabetes. But, good news, West Buffalo Breathers, you are no longer alone. The modern world has now made it possible for you to join a diabetes support group of over 3,000 fellow-sufferers—make that fellow succeeders! The people we're talking about interact with each other 24 hours a day, 7 days a week, by computers through the CompuServe Diabetes and Hypoglycemia Forum. This group is headed up by 46-year-old Dave Groves, who knows whereof he computes because he's had diabetes for 37 years. Not only that, his maternal grandmother became a Type I diabetic 12 years before the discovery of insulin. Her initial therapy consisted of red wine and 500 calories of protein per day. She died of natural causes at the age of 98 with no sign of diabetes complications.

The Forum's charter purpose, Dave says, "is to educate, motivate, and activate diabetics." They do more than that, he explains, including "helping our fellow diabetics to restrain themselves and refrain from punching out the next person who tells them that something like cornsilk tea will prevent complications or that sugar is poison or that there's a cure coming in five years if they will contribute to this, that, or the other fund."

Dave says another major purpose of the forum is "to serve as a sort of computer accessible 'Consumer Reports' regarding diabetes, diabetic products, and diabetic emotions. In this forum," he continues, "you can discuss all aspects of diabetes with other diabetics and experts in the diabetes world from the privacy and comfort of your own home."

According to Dave, in the Forum you'll be on-line with a lot of humor as well. Messages have discussed the aerodynamics of used insulin syringes as darts and bizarre experiences in injecting insulin in public. "People in the Forum," he says, "have a very refreshing attitude!" Some enthusiastic members of the Forum call it "a diabetes summer camp for adults."

The Diabetes Forum has another advantage besides creating a support group for people living in out-of-the way places. It offers people who are in denial or who are embarrassed to go public with their condition a semianonymous way to take the first step. This advantage was pointed out in a *CompuServe Magazine* article about a woman who computer-accessed the "Substance Abuse/AA" section of the Health and Fitness Forum. She asked for information about alcoholism for her husband, whom she described as a problem drinker. After she "attended" a few computerized meetings, it turned out that she was actually the alcoholic in the family but had been unwilling to attend face-to-face meetings. Some of the other people in the forum "talked" to her and encouraged her to go to an AA group in her area. She finally did. She's now chairing an AA beginners group and, as the article stated, "She's doing beautifully."

We asked Dave if he had any recommendations for communication software and modems for people who have computers and are interested in joining the network. Here are his suggestions:

"For people with IBM computers, I highly recommend Crosstalk Communicator with CISOP. It retails for about $40 from your IBM software dealer. For IBM or Mac and rank novices, I would recommend CIM or Navigator (for the Mac). CIM is about $10 from CompuServe, and Navigator 3.0, also available from CompuServe, is just a bit more.

"As far as modems are concerned, Practical Peripherals (1-800-442-4774) has a whole series of good ones from 300 baud to 9600 baud with or without MNP. (A baud is a unit used to measure the speed of electronic data transfer. The higher the baud number, the faster the transfer.) Candidly, I cannot recommend inexpensive modems. The problems they create just serve to frustrate new users and eventually cost them more money. My personal recommendation—not the cheap way—9600 baud with MNP 4.2, but at the very least you should get 2400 baud for file downloading."

The one glitch we've found from our experiences with the CompuServe Diabetes and Hypoglycemia Forum is that it's so fascinating and stimulating that it can be addictive. You have to ration yourself so it doesn't take over your life.

To learn more about CompuServe and the Forum and its monthly fees and hourly rates, you can call: 1-800-848-8199 from anywhere in the United States except Ohio. From Ohio, Canada, Europe, and Australia, call 614-457-0802.

We want to close this chapter with a therapy strategy that hasn't been mentioned yet. We first learned about it back in the 1970s from Dr. Donnell B. Etzwiler, president and chief medical officer of the International Diabetes Center. A pediatric diabetologist practicing at Park Nicollet Medical Center in Minneapolis, Dr. Etzwiler used contracts with his young diabetes patients to help motivate them to take care of themselves. What intrigued us was that some of these contracts had a monetary reward, and that approach seemed to work the best of all with children and teenagers.

Dr. Rubin, it seems to us that contracting could be a useful adjunct to any of the therapies you've talked about. Maybe you could explain contracting and its uses as a kind of generic technique available to anyone working either with a therapist or on his or her own. Incidentally, do you use contracts with your patients? Somehow we suspect that you do.

Dr. Rubin: Your suspicions are confirmed. I use contracts with people I see in my private practice and I use them with the groups I see at Johns Hopkins Diabetes Center. In both settings the approach is similar. Think about what a contract is. It's an agreement to do something in return for something. Good contracts also usually include contingency clauses, statements about what to do if the terms of the contract are in danger of going unmet. And so it goes with the diabetes contracts I have people write. Only there's one essential difference between my contracts and Dr. Etzwiler's: I have people make contracts with themselves, not with me. I think contracts with yourself are the most effective kind. In general, I believe contracts are very helpful for anyone who wants to make changes, diabetes-related or otherwise.

Let me show you how my kind of contracting works. First, as with any contract, I recommend that the agreements embodied in diabetes contracts be put in writing. Cindy Miller, the teaching nurse at the Johns Hopkins Diabetes Center, has used her artistic talents to design an attractive form for the contracts we use there. The form includes three sections: (1) the goals the person agrees to accomplish; (2) the rewards for reaching those goals; and (3) where the person will turn if he or she is slipping. The form is reproduced on the next page.

June and Barbara: That form really makes sense. We can think of lots of ways we could use it ourselves. Since we're first-timers at this, we'd like to have you walk us through it section by section.

Dr. Rubin: With the form in hand, I ask you to answer this question: What would you like to change? Your answer goes in the first section of the contract. I encourage people to be as concrete and specific as possible. This is hard for some people.

MY PERSONAL CONTRACT

Name: _____ Date: _____

I agree to accomplish the following goals:

My rewards for accomplishing these goals are:

If I am in danger of slipping, I will contact:

_____

Signed: _____

For example, someone might say, "I want to exercise more." I'm happy to hear that the person has identified an area for change, but I encourage greater specificity. I might say, "This is a contract. If your boss offered you a contract that said he was going to pay you more, would you be satisfied?" In this day of cutbacks and salary cuts, some people might say yes, but most get my point. They wouldn't be satisfied with that kind of generality. They'd want to know *how much more* they were going to get paid and *when* their raises would come. The same holds true for their diabetes contract. A good exercise goal might sound like this: "I agree to walk 30 minutes three times a week for the next month, then gradually to build up time and pace, as my conditioning permits." That's the ticket, very specific and concrete.

A similar goal for diet might be, "I agree to stop eating all junk food," or "I agree to lose 25 pounds in the next six months." Other concrete goals might include, "I agree to test my blood sugar three times each day," or "I agree to see my doctor every four months," or "I agree to find a good diabetes support group and go to meetings." Get the idea? Specific and concrete.

June and Barbara: Why is it so important to be specific and concrete?

Dr. Rubin: Because it's been demonstrated time and again that this is the kind of goal successful people set for themselves. It's easier to achieve goals you can visualize. Once you're reached such a goal, you're highly motivated to set your next goal. And so it goes, onward and upward, one day and one goal at a time.

June and Barbara: We're true believers in that kind of goal-setting. Do you have any cautions and warnings about mistakes we might make when we set out to set our goals?

Dr. Rubin: Yes. First, the goals must be ones you really want to reach. This might sound ridiculously obvious, but I think it's not. Goals that are your doctor's or your spouse's but not your own are unachievable. You'll never reach them. That doesn't mean you can't have the same goals as those who care for you; it just means that you must be crystal-clear that the goal you identify is yours first and foremost.

In addition, your goals should be realistically ambitious. If you set a goal that is way beyond your capacities, you'll soon lose heart and tear up your contract. If, for example, you set a goal of losing 150 pounds in six months or of testing your blood eight times every day, you're setting yourself up for disappointment. If, on the other hand, you set a goal that requires no stretch at all—losing five pounds in the next year when you're 100 pounds overweight, say, or testing your blood once a week when you're taking insulin—you aren't going to get much from your contract either.

You can specify several steps toward the ultimate accomplishment of your goal, with the number of steps determined by how far you are from your goal. Start where you are and build slowly and steadily. Let's say you're currently doing no exercise and you're in pretty poor condition. Start with a modest exercise program until you get comfortable with it, then gradually increase it. You'll be amazed how far you can go with this approach. This attitude also applies to the number of goals you set. Start with one or two things that matter most to you. That will get you rolling and feeling successful. Then you can go from there. Today a 30-minute walk, tomorrow the world, right?

June and Barbara: Right! Now we're ready for the fun part of the contract, the rewards. It sounds easy to decide to do something nice for yourself, but there's probably a best way to do even that.

Dr. Rubin: It is a little trickier than it seems. You have to start by deciding what you really find rewarding. This might sound obvious, but it's really important. We want to help you find all the motivation you can, and motivation is strongest when the rewards are really rewarding. Rewards come in all shapes and sizes: feeling more energetic (for reaching a goal of better blood sugars), feeling proud (for taking good care of yourself), a new wardrobe (for losing 30 pounds and finding that nothing in your closet fits you anymore), a longer, healthier life (for reaching all your goals), a trip down the Amazon River (this last one was mentioned by one participant in a Diabetes Center course). Those suggestions ought to stimulate your thinking. What rewards do you seek? People often identify a mix of health-related, emotional, and material rewards, and that seems like a good mix for maximum motivation.

June and Barbara: We realize the path toward our contractual goal is strewn with banana peels. How do we keep ourselves from slipping up?

Dr. Rubin: You may need someone to help you over the risky places. For relapse protection think of those people you can really count on. How about your doctor, your nurse-educator (if you're fortunate enough to have one), your spouse, a good friend, someone you know who has diabetes, or a support group? Any of these can help. To whom you turn is not important; having *someone* to whom you can turn is. The time to identify that person or those persons is now, not later when you really need them. Later you will not be thinking clearly. You might also forewarn the person and explain the kind of help you think you might need.

Last, but certainly not least, when it comes to relapse protectors, don't forget your Sympathetic Scientist. If all else fails, sit down with your contract and your SS and see what help that inner adviser can provide. I guarantee you'll get something useful to work on.

June and Barbara: One last thing. After you've written up your contract, what do you do with it?

Dr. Rubin: Put it up on your refrigerator, on your bathroom mirror, or over your bed—any place where you'll see it often and be reminded of the goals you set, the reward you promised yourself, and the sources of support you identified when you were at your best. I've found that these diabetes contracts can work wonderfully. Do one with your health-care provider or do one on your own, but do one.

➤ Help for Those Who Want to Help Diabetics

June and Barbara: There is a woman we care about, now in her 80s, who's always lived an extremely active life with lots of socializing with friends and extensive travel (she's been to China four times). A couple of years ago she had a serious heart attack, then, not long afterward, a fall that caused recurrent back pain, and finally hip surgery that left her with one leg shorter than the other, making walking difficult. While recuperating from the broken hip she became extremely depressed because she began to realize that her active life was going to be extremely curtailed. She has given up driving. Her depression continues to deepen, and she's even been making hints about suicide.

We suggested to her that she should have some therapy to help her through this period. She flatly refused. The reasons she gave were: "I'm a very private person" (that's certainly true) and "I don't like those people," meaning anyone in the field of psychology or psychiatry. The words "those people" were delivered with the derisive inflection a prejudiced person would use if members of a detested racial or ethnic group moved into the neighborhood.

We know from what you've said that nobody can make anyone else do something they don't want to do. So, since we're not capable of giving her any kind of effective counsel ourselves, do we just let her sit there in her sink of depression? Is there something we can do to get her to want to go to a therapist? Can you suggest something else that might help us and, more important, help those who are trying to get a reluctant diabetic to go into needed counseling?

Dr. Rubin: It is my experience that counseling does no good unless the patient wants it. That doesn't mean that doctors, family, and friends should stand idly by as the diabetic slowly slides into emotional oblivion. Not for a moment. They should suggest, encourage, even cajole the prospective counselee. These efforts might help the diabetic find his or her own motivation to seek treatment, but they can't provide that motivation for the diabetic. That's a painful fact, but a fact nonetheless.

Once the skeptical diabetic is sitting in the same room as the therapist, it's part of the therapist's job to help the patient locate his or her motivation for change. But again, the therapist can't provide that motivation.

As you point out, denying an apparent need for therapy is like denying the reality of diabetes, or in your friend's case the reality of the accumulated health problems that sent her into depression. This kind of denial is obviously self-destructive, and it is extremely frustrating for anyone who loves, lives with, or cares for the denying person. What you have to do is recognize, grieve, and finally accept the reality of your own limits to help. You should never stop trying new ways of helping the person locate his or her motivation for change. Asking your loved one if there's any way you might help to bring about the result might be a good idea. But in the final analysis you just have to let go of the expectation that the person you care about will change and seek counseling because you feel that is the answer.

POSITIVE FRAMING
SWIMMING TO BORA BORA

As we were finishing this book, Dr. Rubin came up with a good analysis of what we've tried to do. The negative emotion chapters are about keeping yourself from drowning—learning how to stay afloat in your life with diabetes. The therapy chapter is about getting outside help if you're having trouble keeping your head above water. This final chapter is about swimming.

Now that you've reached this point, you have an important decision to make. Let's pretend you're paddling around in the waters of the South Pacific in an area a little to the north of Tahiti. In one direction is a bare coral atoll—no coconut palms, no fresh water, no life, no nothing. In the opposite direction, about the same distance away, is Bora Bora—an island James Michener described as the most beautiful place on the face of the earth. He used it as a model for his book *Tales of the South Pacific*. The island's beaches are of soft white sand. Walk out a little way into the warm, clear turquoise water, put on your snorkeling mask, float face-down and you can see the flashing colors of the most varied collection of tropical fish anywhere in the world.

On shore you have a comfortable grass hut with a lazily turning ceiling fan. Outside your door are lush green plants with flame-colored flowers, and a hammock where you can rest, read, dream, and contemplate the changing cloud formations in the cerulean sky. When you're hungry you can find an abundance of wonderful French cuisine with tropical touches and warm, loving people to enjoy it with. There's music and dancing and laughter. It is, in short, Paradise. To which island do you swim?

That seems like a ridiculous question, doesn't it? Anyone in their right mind would swim to Bora Bora. Unfortunately, that's not always true. Many people in their right minds don't even realize they have a choice. For some reason they think there's only one direction they can swim: to the bare, lifeless atoll, and this they grimly do, day after day after day. Others are almost as bad off, spending their whole lives treading water, not knowing which way to go.

All of us swim in the wrong direction and tread water from time to time. But it doesn't have to be. We can change, and it's not as difficult to do as you may think.

Dr. Rubin will now jump into the water, point us in the right direction, and give us a personal swimming lesson. We'll meet you a little later on Bora Bora.

—June and Barbara

June and Barbara: This chapter, Dr. Rubin, is all yours. We're going to sit back quietly while you teach us how to make our lives with diabetes beautiful using the methods you've worked out and perfected during your career as brother of, father of, and therapist for diabetics.

Dr. Rubin: That's a big order, but I feel up to the challenge and I love having the opportunity. Opportunity, in fact, is the key word here. In the Chinese language the word for crisis is made up of two separate characters. One means disaster; the other, opportunity. The chapters about negative emotions were intended to help you keep your diabetes from becoming a disaster. This one is to help you turn your diabetes into an opportunity.

Does this sound like pie in the sky? Maybe you can accept the idea that there are ways to keep diabetes from overwhelming you, but seeing your disease as an opportunity—that's too much. I can understand your skepticism. Bear with me and I think I can convince you of the plausibility and the power of this perspective.

Let me start with a story that appeared in *Parade,* the Sunday newspaper insert, in August 1988. The story was about Marie Ragghianti, the heroine of the book and movie *Marie.* Marie had risked her livelihood by exposing corruption in the Tennessee state government for which she worked. Marie explains in the article that the greatest influence on her life was her mother. At the age of 31 her mother had been left paralyzed by a spinal tumor. A vibrant woman who could do anything, overnight she became confined to a wheelchair. Although she could no longer do many of the things she had before, she faced her illness with the same enthusiasm she had brought to everything before the confinement.

When Marie was grown and entered the field of corrections (she eventually became chairman of Tennessee's Board of Pardons and Paroles), her mother became interested in working with prisoners. She taught creative writing to inmates until she could no longer go out to the prison; then she began corresponding with several prisoners. One day she asked Marie to mail a letter to a prisoner. Marie asked to read it first, and it was a great revelation to her. Here is the letter:

Dear Waymon:
I want you to know that I have been thinking about you often since receiving your letter. You mentioned how difficult it is to be locked behind bars, and my heart goes out to you. But when you said I couldn't imagine what it is like to be in prison, I felt impelled to tell you that you are mistaken.

There are different kinds of freedom, Waymon, different kinds of prisons. Sometimes our prisons are self-imposed.

When at the age of 31, I awoke one day to find that I was completely paralyzed, I felt trapped—overwhelmed by a sense of being imprisoned in a body that would no longer allow me to run through a meadow or dance or carry my child in my arms . . .

I thought about this concept of imprisonment, because it seemed to me that I had lost everything in life that mattered. I was near despair. But then one day it occurred to me that, in fact, there were still some options open to me and that I had the freedom to choose among them . . .

I made a decision to strive, as long as I was alive, to live as fully as I could, to seek to turn my seemingly negative experiences into positive experiences, to look for ways to transcend my physical limitations by expanding my mental and spiritual boundaries . . .

You can look at your bars, or you can look through them . . . To some extent, Waymon, we are in this thing together.

What made it possible for this woman to be so strong; to go beyond simply coping with her disability to transcending it? You might say she had tremendous inner resources, and I'd agree. You might admire this woman; who wouldn't? You might even stand in awe of her; I know that I do. But you might also feel that you could never aspire to her capacities. To this I say, "nonsense." In support of my position I quote that great sage, Dr. Seuss, from his book *Oh, the Places You'll Go!:*

> You have brains in your head,
> You have feet in your shoes.
> You can steer yourself
> In any direction you choose.

Listen to what the good doctor is saying. The key to the kind of transcendence Marie Ragghianti's mother achieved is attitude. Her attitude created the kind of positive self-fulfilling prophecy I talked about in earlier chapters. Attitude is not something you're born with. It's a skill you develop. No one is born with a positive attitude (or a negative one, for that matter) any more than anyone is born able to operate a computer, knit a sweater, or drive a car.

How do you develop the skill of a positive attitude? There are two steps, and they are simple but not easy. First, you have to use your head (and your heart) to set your goal. ("You have brains in your head.") Then, you have to practice, with patience and perseverance, as you get closer and closer to your goal. ("You have feet in your shoes.") This might sound like a pretty tall order, and it is. But you're already doing exactly what I've described, at least every once in a while. Let me prove it to you.

Think about the situation that bugs you most day-to-day about your diabetes. Maybe it's finding the time to test your blood in the morning with all the rushing around you have to do. Or maybe you can't resist grazing after dinner. Or maybe you find it almost impossible to exercise as you should. Whatever your particular biggest bugaboo, see if you can remember an occasion (even if it was only once) when things went a little easier than usual, a time when you were able to do the right thing without feeling quite so upset or overwhelmed. If you're like most people, you can remember at least a few such instances.

What do you think was different about those times? Let's say the problem is grazing. You might say, "I was out of the house," or "I ate so much for dinner that I just wasn't interested." That makes sense to me, because circumstances do have an effect. But wasn't there an evening when you were home and you hadn't overeaten at dinner but still managed to pass on the grazing? Almost certainly you'll answer yes to this question, if you think about it for a while.

What do you think accounted for your success on that occasion? Probably something about your attitude or frame of mind. So you do know how to "Steer yourself in any direction you choose." You just don't know how to do it consistently. Even so, you're already living proof that the Greek philosopher Epictetus was right when he wrote that we are disturbed

not by things, but by the view we take of them. I could para-
phrase that positively by saying that we are not *inspired* by
things, but by the view we take of them.

The major trick is to use what I call positive frames to create a mood where something good can happen. This something good means taking care of yourself physically and emotionally as far as your diabetes is concerned and every other
aspect of your life. Over the years I've discovered a number of
positive frames to choose from, and each is a perspective
guaranteed to create that something-good-can-happen mood.
The frames have to be positive, because it's the frame of a picture that defines the meaning of what's in the picture. You
want to turn all your negative pictures of diabetes into positive
ones. I find the seven most effective frames are: the frame of
partializing, the frame of letting go, the frame of love, the
frame of faith and hope, the frame of humor, the frame of sharing information, and finally the frame of celebration. I know
you've never heard of these. My colleague Dr. Joseph Napora
and I worked them out together over a long period and we
both use them successfully to help people find attitudes that
create positive happenings in their lives. You may invent other
frames to put around diabetes situations to bring about a
happy result.

There's a childhood song we all know that offers a perfect
prescription for creating a mood where something good can
happen. It illustrates perfectly the principle on which positive
framing works:

> Row, row, row your boat,
> Gently down the stream.
> Merrily, merrily, merrily, merrily,
> Life is but a dream.

Listen to what the rhyme tells us. "Row, row, row your
boat": this says that life, in general and with diabetes in particular, is work. But that work should be undertaken "gently
down [not up] the stream." In other words, go with the flow.

And we should go about our business "merrily," to further assure a good mood. Finally, we are reminded of a fundamental truth: "Life is but a dream." We create its meaning, and we can make that meaning wonderful or horrible. The choice is ours.

How do you make the choice for wonderful? You use positive frames. I'll tell you a story that will help you see exactly how positive frames work in specific situations.

A substitute teacher was writing on the blackboard, innocent of the fact that her students had conspired to get her goat by each pushing a book onto the floor while her back was turned. At the sudden thunderous crash, the teacher wheeled around to see the class all looking at her, innocent as babes. She knew what they were up to, and she quickly assessed her options—her frames. She felt challenged, maybe even threatened, and she could have responded by punishing the class and keeping everyone after school. This would almost certainly *not* have created a mood where something good could happen, for the students or for her. Another option was to ignore the challenge. She could have turned around and gone back to her writing. But kids being kids, the provocations would probably have escalated until they would have been impossible to ignore, so that didn't seem like a viable option for creating a good mood, either. Then the teacher realized she had a third frame available. She walked over to her desk, knocked a book onto the floor, and said, "Sorry I'm late." The tension broke, the students laughed, retrieved their books, and went back to their lesson.

The teacher found a positive frame in this situation, one that definitely created a mood where something good could happen. But in order to get there she had to resist a strong temptation to frame the situation negatively and to react impulsively in a way that would create a mood where something bad was almost certain to happen. This is a key point: to frame positively and create a positive mood, you must almost always resist a natural impulse. You must, as my colleague Dr. Napora likes to put it, pull the plug on your jukebox. We are all programmed like jukeboxes. Someone presses a particular button and we play a particular tune. That's what we have to resist. Because that particular tune is probably creating a bad mood, not a good one, or we wouldn't be having a problem in the first place.

Olympic athletes are the personification of positive framing. They imagine feats of physical grace and endurance no one has ever performed, and then they set out to perform them. Sometimes their progress is very slow, and often they never achieve their ultimate goal, and yet they persevere. They must constantly work against the natural human tendency to give up in the face of gigantic challenge. Some positive frame carries them on against the odds. Even in the face of apparent defeat they do not yield. They must be recognizing the possibility for a victory invisible to all but themselves.

I felt this strongly as I watched the figure skating in the 1988 Winter Olympics. The competition for the gold medal was so intense that even one modest slip meant the end of a skater's hopes. As several of the top performers made such slips, I marveled at their ability to continue their routines. "Why don't they just skate off the ice?" I asked myself. "Can't they see they've lost the competition?" Slowly it dawned on me that while they had lost the medal, they hadn't lost the competition, because the true competition was within the skater, and it encompassed all the competitions to come, as well.

When you have diabetes you need to be an Olympic athlete of positive framing. The skill is essential to truly living well with your disease. Once you've developed that skill, you can apply it to every area of your life. Here are my seven positive frames you can begin using. I'll tell you about each of them along with some stories about how they work.

THE FRAME OF PARTIALIZING
One of the big problems people have in living with diabetes is the fact that everything seems so complicated. Sometimes a situation may look like an insurmountable mountain, totally blocking your path toward a desired outcome. Positive framing by partializing starts with the question, "How can I break this

problem down into manageable pieces so I can create a mood where something good can happen?" Here's an example, provided by one of my patients, Gail.

Gail was leaving work one evening when several of her friends suggested she join them for a light supper before going home. She immediately said no, because she didn't have her insulin with her, she had to pick up her preschool-age son at day care, and her husband would be home expecting dinner. As she drove home she felt angry and depressed: "Damned diabetes, damned life. I can never do anything fun. There's always a thousand things that make it impossible. Grumble, grumble, grumble."

She was working herself into a good funk, when she remembered the frame of partializing, which we had talked about the day before. She stopped her negative self-talk and asked herself how she could have broken down the "impossible" problem into manageable chunks. "Well," she said to herself, "I could have suggested that we go to that restaurant near my house. Then I could have called my husband and told him to pick up a pizza for himself and Timmy. I know he wouldn't have minded. I could have gotten Timmy at day care and left him with my neighbor for 15 minutes until my husband got home. Then I could have taken my shot and been to the restaurant about 20 minutes after my friends. They'd be eating appetizers first anyway, and I'm better off skipping them. That would all have taken some doing, but when I look at it a piece at a time, it's manageable. And it's worlds better than feeling left out and deprived."

Partializing does take thought and planning, as well as resisting that initial impulse to say, "No. It's impossible." This one-step-at-a-time, one-day-at-a-time approach also works for longer-term projects like improving blood-sugar control or establishing a healthy exercise program. These tasks can seem overwhelming when they're viewed monolithically, so don't look at them that way. Find a way to break them down into manageable, bite-sized chunks. Set your long-term goal and then set monthly, weekly, or even daily goals as stepping-stones. I know a diabetic woman who runs 50- and 100-mile races. (This is not a misprint. I do mean miles!) Ten years ago she took her first step toward this achievement. She ran from her front door to the corner, a distance of half a block. She arrived at her destination out of breath, but convinced that all she had to do was keep it up, day after day. She was right.

The one-day-at-a-time approach in pursuit of a lofty goal reminds me of how I worked on my Ph.D. dissertation 20 years ago. I knew this was going to be a huge undertaking, I knew that I would have essentially no direction except what I provided myself, and I knew that other people going through this process spent much of their time panicked, spinning their wheels, or working insane hours. What was I going to do? I drew on my experience as a factory worker, a job I had held for three summers during high school and college. Why I did this I still cannot say, but it turned out to be a real inspiration. I decided that if I got to my work cubicle at exactly 8:00 every morning Monday through Friday, worked until exactly noon, took exactly 30 minutes for lunch and socializing, and then worked until exactly 5:00 P.M., I could completely forget about the dissertation after 5:00 each weekday and for the entire weekend. Sounds kind of weird, doesn't it? On certain mornings it looked weird, as I ran to the library in order to "punch in" on time at my cubicle.

Weird it might have been, but it worked. I stayed calm, which is more than I could say for the vast majority of my peers who were undertaking the same rite of passage. I had all this wonderful dissertation-free time. Day by day and week by week, the pile of finished manuscript pages steadily mounted, until finally I was done. I had broken down my problem into a series of manageable daylong chunks and succeeded in creating a mood where something good could happen—and it did.

THE FRAME OF LETTING GO
When you have diabetes, it's often hard to let go of certain unrealistic expectations. "I don't really have to deal with this

disease," for instance, or "I have to do everything perfectly." Refusing to let go is like banging your head against a brick wall. The wall won't budge, but you'll end up with a sore head and a badly bruised ego. Letting go does not mean giving up; it means living by the words of the Serenity Prayer I keep referring to: "Grant me the serenity to accept the things I cannot change, the courage to change the things I can, and the wisdom to know the difference." Letting go means protecting your precious energy and resources for battles you can win, rather than wasting them on ones you can't. The key to positive framing through letting go is answering the question, "What do I need to let go of so I can create a mood where something good can happen?"

I'm reminded of Itzhak Perlman, the renowned violinist, who had polio as a child. As a result of this disease, Perlman has no use of his legs. When he performs, he makes his way onstage using crutches, and someone places his violin next to his chair. He gave an interview a few years ago in which he said that he realized at a young age that he didn't need his legs to do the thing that was most important to him in life— play the violin. The lesson he lives by is, "Don't pay attention to what doesn't work. That's a waste of time. Pay attention to what does work." I'm sure there are times when Perlman feels sad about his disability. Letting go is a painful process, because it involves accepting the loss of something precious. No one can do that without tears and anger. But, as we talked about in the Grieving chapter, letting go is an essential part of healing. If we don't let go, we can't move on. When you have diabetes, letting go is a daily challenge. Everyone makes mistakes; no one is perfect. And perfect control of diabetes is impossible to achieve, as we've said so often. When you make a mistake or get a blood sugar that upsets you, try to learn from the experience, and then let go so you can move on. Don't hang on to disappointed feelings, and don't keep trying the same things over and over when they don't work. Stop beating your head against the wall. As W. C. Fields once said, "If at first you don't succeed, try again. Then quit. There's no use being a damn fool about it."

As I write, two personal experiences stand out in my mind for their power as lessons in the importance of letting go. One was almost trivial, the other anything but. I'll tell the trivial story first. I used to live in a city rowhouse in a friendly neighborhood where I enjoyed sitting in my backyard chatting with friends and acquaintances up and down the block. The pleasures of the backyard grew after I created a wonderful little garden there. Sitting among my greenery and flowers, gazing up and down the row of other yards felt heavenly. Then one day I came home from work in the early evening, stepped out my back door to settle into my little world, only to be confronted by the ugliest, highest wooden fence I'd ever seen, put up that day by my nextdoor neighbor. My beautiful garden was now bordered by this hideous wall, and my view of all the backyards on that side was gone forever. I was furious and miserable. I could no longer enjoy my yard.

I was so preoccupied by my loss that at first I didn't notice the gorgeous butterfly that circled my head in the growing dusk. It circled again and again, so close I could almost touch it, until at last it caught my attention. It fluttered out into the garden and landed on the most beautiful blossom of my favorite peony bush. It stayed there until I got the message: "You can stare at the fence and make yourself miserable, or you can gaze on me and the peony. Where do you choose to focus?"

The other experience is my hardest letting-go ever. For 15 years I was married to Kay (Stefan's mom). We married fairly young (I was 25 and Kay was 22), and I felt our life together was the greatest gift I had ever received. Every day I would bounce up the steps when I came home from work. I was that excited to see Kay. We shared so much that I felt I was truly in a state of grace.

Then in the summer of 1983, Kay met another person and fell deeply in love. So deeply, in fact, that she had no choice but to leave me. The end of our relationship was very sudden and very final. I was devastated, hurt, and angry almost beyond bearing. I did my best to maintain a civil relationship with Kay for the sake of the children, but I was not always successful. My pain and rage often spilled over and out. For several years

I could not let go of these feelings. I could not accept what had happened. As a result, I couldn't heal, and I couldn't move on.

Slowly, by stops and starts, I did heal. I found the serenity to accept the thing I could not change, the fact that my marriage with Kay was over, and perhaps more painful than that, the fact that my sense of our marriage had been in part a fantasy. But with the letting go came a gift—the courage to change what I could. I found that I could reclaim what had always been truest in my relationship with Kay: a wonderful friendship. We are today, and I hope will always be, among each other's deepest friends.

Letting go was not easy. It is not completely easy even now, years later. In fact, tears are flowing as I write. But tears are balm for the soul, and my heart is strong and full. I have let go and I have healed.

THE FRAME OF LOVE

Feelings of fear, resentment, and isolation are all common when you live with diabetes. These emotions can undermine everyone's physical and emotional health. When you answer the question, "How can I reach out with love and create a mood where something good can happen?" you use the frame of love to do battle against hopelessness and isolation. You create the strength together with your loved one to deal with the problems you face.

I mentioned earlier that there was a period before Stefan got his insulin pump when he would take what seemed forever pushing the needle of the syringe into his flesh. He would sit there with the needle poised for minutes at a time, and I often felt irritated, occasionally exhorting him to just get it over with and arguing that his approach actually increased his pain. Not surprisingly, he found this impatient advice unhelpful, and to tell the truth, I didn't feel too great about it, either.

I tried to come up with a new tack, starting with how I actually felt. Once I looked within, I realized that the irritation I felt was a cover for deeper feelings: love for my son and sadness that he had to endure the shots that so obviously pained him. The next morning as he began his slow-motion ritual, I said, "I know those shots hurt like hell. I even get a knot in my stomach when you stick yourself. I would give anything to be able to take some of them for you. You're really brave, and I love you, love you, love you." Stefan looked at me with a little smile on his lips and said, "It's not *that* big a deal." With that he pushed the needle right in.

A patient told me, "I was diagnosed four months ago, and the diabetes has actually brought my wife and me closer. We walk miles every day and talk and talk. I think the dog likes the walks, too, though I'm afraid we've about worn her paws to nothing."

When someone close to you gets angry over some diabetes-related issue, it feels terrible. How can they act that way if they care about you? The fact is, their behavior isn't the result of a lack of love. They may care so much that they're over-whelmed by their fears for you and the responsibility they feel for your well-being. It's not easy to do, but it can really help if you're able to see through their anger to the deep love and caring underneath. This can help because you'll feel less iso-lated, and you can respond with love yourself, rather than de-fensively. You might even be so bold as to say, "I can tell you're really concerned for me, and I love you for it. I don't know what I'd do without you." This kind of statement has the power to stop a negative interaction dead in its tracks, and maybe even turn it around, transforming it into something new and potentially wonderful.

It goes without saying that you need to love yourself. That's hard for most of us, but, as someone once told me, "I'm the only person I'll have to wake up with every morning of my life, so I better start being nice to myself." Sound advice. An-other patient said, "I've been trying to deal with my fears by getting my family together to talk about my diabetes. I tell them that I always thought I was the sweetest one in the fam-ily, and now I know I am."

Consulting your Sympathetic Scientist can help here. The better you feel about yourself, the easier you'll find it to create a mood where something good can happen. One way to help this process along is, before you go to sleep at night, to tell yourself three things you did during the day that you feel good about. If this sounds silly, let me assure you that, silly or not, it's effective. So are many other ways to love yourself. Make time for things that bring you true pleasure and for people with whom you feel really good. Bottom line: cherish yourself. No one deserves it more, and no one can do it better.

THE FRAME OF FAITH AND HOPE

Faith and hope can be a solid barrier against the tide of diabetes-related emotional pain. Answer the question, What are my sources of faith, and how can I draw on them to create a mood where something good can happen? This is your first step to positive framing through faith and hope. Different people have different sources for their faith. For some, faith in a higher power is a tremendous source of strength. Other people draw mostly on faith in their family and friends or in themselves.

One man expressed his faith in himself this way: "I was diagnosed six weeks ago. I don't see diabetes as an incredible liability, even though I work as a chef and I'm used to cooking and eating things made with butter and heavy cream and such. Now I have to change all that and get into healthy eating and exercise. I see diabetes as a kind of kick in the butt in these areas. I feel confident and positive."

Others have faith in their capacity to deal with diabetes because they've coped with other diseases. Still others are sustained by hope for a better future. Most often this hope is provided by the rapid advances in medical science and technology. I see this source of faith most strongly among kids with diabetes and their parents. Sometimes the way the kids express themselves is very poignant. I was talking with a group of 10-to-12-year-olds about what it would be like if a cure were found for diabetes. A rapturous expression came over the face of one boy, and he said, "It would be like I was in *The Sound of Music.*"

Sometimes faith can be too strong. A few years ago I was working with a family whose 4-year-old son had just been diagnosed with diabetes. They seemed to be adjusting well, and they all became very involved in the Juvenile Diabetes Foundation's annual Walk to Cure Diabetes. The most active of all was the little boy. He canvassed his neighborhood for contributions, called every relative asking for pledges, and swore that he would walk the entire 10 kilometers under his own power—no carrying for him. His parents and I were amazed at his dedication.

Sure enough, the boy walked the entire distance, and then religiously collected all his pledges within the next couple of days. He insisted on going with his mother to turn in the impressive total he had earned. That night, as his mother was tucking him into bed, he asked, "Will I be cured before I wake up tomorrow?" He had taken the slogan of the march literally, and he had certainly done his part.

That reminds me of a story, apocryphal, I'm sure. A small Midwestern town was deluged by rain for days. The streets began to fill with water, and the townspeople started to evacuate. In the middle of town stood a church, and the flood waters had reached its doors. A boat approached as the priest stood at the top of the steps, up to his ankles in water. "We've got to get you out," a man in the boat called, "it's not safe." "No," the priest replied, "the Lord will provide." The next day the waters were up to the second story of the church, and another boat approached, imploring the priest to get aboard. "No," he answered again, "the Lord will provide." By the next day the flood had covered the entire church except for the steeple, to which the priest clung. Once again a boat approached. The man in the boat said, "I'm the last one in town except for you. Climb in now!" "No," the priest intoned, "the Lord will provide."

By the next day the church was completely under water and the priest had been swept away and drowned. The moment he arrived in heaven he sought out God. When he found God, he said, "With all due respect, Lord, I'm a little disappointed. I clung to my faith that you would provide and you let me down." "Let you down?" God retorted. "I sent you three boats, didn't I?"

The moral here is that God helps those who help themselves. Faith is a vehicle, and a very powerful one at that, for creating a better life. But you have to participate in the creation.

THE FRAME OF HUMOR

The two closest things to magic in this world are faith and humor. If you can use them both to frame positively, your success is almost guaranteed. Answering the question, How can I use humor to create a mood where something good can happen? can have truly liberating consequences. Laughter feels good. I've read descriptions of humor as "internal jogging" that helps you relax and relieve feelings of frustration and disappointment just as physical exercise does.

You may think I've gone off the deep end. Laughter and diabetes? But so often people who have gone through a traumatic experience say they couldn't have made it without a sense of humor. Here are a couple of non-diabetes-related examples, both true stories. A woman was in the hospital for breast cancer surgery. When the orderlies came to wheel her to the operating room, she was wearing a propeller beanie, and she had a big colorful sign on her chest that said, "Give it your best shot." A note attached to the sign read, "Do not remove this sign until the surgeon sees it." When the operating room nurse asked what she was doing, she replied, "When that surgeon cuts me today, I want him to be in a good mood."

Another woman drove her car off a bridge, plunging into the river below. She tried to force open the doors, but the water pressure made that impossible. She managed to get her head up into a little air pocket at the top of the car and was on the verge of panic, when she noticed that various items from her pocketbook were bobbing by her nose. First her wallet, then her lipstick, then an old lottery ticket. The scene was so absurd that she actually laughed, which eased her fear, and she lived to tell the tale.

My own first diabetes-related experience with the healing power of humor came on the day that Stefan was diagnosed. Sitting in the pediatrician's office, feeling almost as bad as I could imagine feeling, I heard Dr. Bill ask me to pull down my pants and stick myself with a syringe to show Stefan that it wasn't overwhelmingly painful. As bad as I felt, an absurd thought crossed my mind, "At least I'm wearing clean underwear" (just as mother always advised me). After I had complied with Bill's request, he asked Kay to do the same. We'd been friends with the doctor for so long that this seemed completely natural. Down came Kay's pants to reveal another pair of my clean underwear. Apparently, she'd run out of her own and decided to use a pair of mine. Somehow, the ridiculousness of the whole scene raised my spirits a notch or two.

One basic key to framing with humor is to carry the kind of exaggerated thinking that makes a situation distressful to its illogical and often hilarious conclusion. Here's an experience I had with Stefan that illustrates this approach. Stefan did beautifully with his diabetes for the first couple of years, until he had to start taking a shot at dinnertime in addition to the one he had always taken at breakfast. For some reason, this shot was his Waterloo. Every evening after the regimen changed he would ask angrily or beseechingly, "Why do I have to take the second shot? Why can't I just take one shot a day?" Thinking he was asking for information, I drew him a graph, illustrating insulin action and food action to show why the extra shot was important. This was absolutely no help in easing his resistance. Weeks went by with Stefan's screaming escalating and me doggedly drawing more and more elaborate graphs, somehow blindly convinced that somewhere there was a diagram that would end our confrontation. No such luck.

Finally, one evening my son asked his nightly question, "Why can't I take just one shot a day?" and I froze, just as I was about to draw yet another graph. A light bulb went on in my head just like the ones you see in the cartoons. I looked at him and said, "Sounds good to me, but wouldn't you rather have one shot a week?" He looked at me in amazement for a moment before his own light bulb went on. Then he asked, "How about one shot a month?" To which I replied, now fully in the spirit, "Let's go for the whole ball of wax. Make it one shot a year." We both laughed. Then Stefan's eyes clouded up and he said, "But think about how big the syringe would have to be!" He quickly multiplied his daily dose by the number of days in a year and came up with 12,775 units of insulin. One hell of a syringe! We both laughed again. That night Stefan took his shot without complaint, which was a great relief. But my biggest surprise was to come the next night, and the next, and the next: he never asked the question again.

I believe that Stefan was never asking me about that second shot. What he was really saying, though he didn't know how to express it directly, was, "This second shot is the straw that broke the camel's back. I'm overwhelmed and I need your help lightening the load." When I finally got the message and responded to it instinctively, I solved our problem and learned an important lesson in the bargain. When someone is struggling unsuccessfully with a diabetes-related issue (or even a non-diabetes-related issue, for that matter), the key to success is to lighten the emotional load by any means that work, including humor. Once the load has been lightened, you can deal with the issue much more easily, because the fundamental problem is not the issue itself, but the sense of being overwhelmed. It's important to keep in mind that the purpose of framing with humor is not to ignore or deny a serious situation, but simply to lower the level of emotional tension so the situation can be dealt with constructively.

Sometimes the situation you must deal with constructively is a chronic one. Here, too, humor can help. A blind woman was in counseling to help improve her emotional coping skills. Among the things she found to help herself was riding her exercise bike, often for hours at a time. One day during a counseling session, her therapist, with whom she had developed a very comfortable relationship, jokingly suggested that she get a real bike and take it for a spin around her neighborhood. The woman laughed, then added, "But if I did that I would only experience the few blocks around my house. When I ride my exercise bike, I can go anywhere in the world."

Thinking of blind diabetics reminds me of the talking blood-testing meters that are now available, and of a great new marketing idea my colleague Joseph Napora and I came up with. We liked the idea of a talking meter so much that we thought, "Hey, why should we have them only for people who can't see? How about a whole range of talking meters available for everybody?"

First off, the little computer chip could be personalized to say your name. Even better, you could buy one that talked to you the way you wanted to be talked to. For instance, imagine that your Sympathetic Scientist was programmed into your meter. Let's say you had a reading of 317 mg/dl (17.6 mmol/L). The meter would say, "Hmm, looks like a 317, Sam, that's higher than usual for you at 7:12 A.M. Let's see if we can figure out what caused it, and where we go from here. Don't worry too much. We're experts at this kind of detective work. And your blood sugars have been really good recently. Your average for the last two weeks is 164 mg/dl (9.1 mmol/L), so one high one every once in a while isn't that serious. Anyway, let's see what we can come up with."

Or you might prefer a Pushy Prosecutor model. This one might say: "A 317! I knew it! Okay, I want to hear everything you've done since your last test, and I mean *everything*. Don't even try to lie to me, because I'll get the truth out of you, if it's the last thing I do." Or maybe you'd prefer a Guilt Getter model that takes an approach like this: "Oh, so you're finally testing again. This is only the second time you've done that in the last three weeks. Do you have any idea of the damage you could be doing to your body? And imagine what your doctor will say when you go for your next appointment with almost no readings." How about a meter that's programmed to provide the ultimate in user friendliness: "Hi, Sally. Gosh, it's great to see you again. Hope everything's going well. The kids? The dog? Well, let's see what the number is today. 158. Not bad at all. So what are you planning for breakfast? Okay, take care of yourself. Have a good, healthy day. You're a really sweet person, and a good one, too. See you tonight."

As you can see, the possibilities are endless. Until these meters are a reality you can pretend you have one by talking to yourself when you test. Just decide what you'd like to hear your meter say and imagine that it's saying it.

I hear some great stories when I give talks to groups of diabetics and their loved ones. Here are a couple of my favorites. One man told me that he had just been diagnosed. After his doctor gave him all the basic information about his disease and its treatment, the man said, "I understand it could affect my sex life." "Let me put it to you this way," his doctor responded. "If your blood sugars go up, you don't."

A woman said that she had had a reaction the night before a talk I gave. She was too shaky to go downstairs for food, so her husband went to fetch a sandwich and juice. She waited and waited for him to return. When he finally did, he was empty-handed. "Where's my sandwich and juice?" the woman demanded indignantly. "Oh, my God," her husband responded. "I ate them."

"Fine," you might be saying at this point. "I can see that humor really can create a mood where something good can happen, but I'm no stand-up comic. I'm just not that fast on my feet. In fact, I can hardly even remember jokes I've heard." No problem, you don't need to be. Humor is everywhere. You just need to discover it in the situations where it automatically pops up and to remember it in situations where you really need it.

THE FRAME OF SHARING INFORMATION

This frame is based on the necessity of communication with those around you in order to create that mood (on everybody's part) where something good can happen. After all, people can't read your mind, nor you theirs. When you believe otherwise, you almost always take a big risk of creating a mood where something *bad* is likely to happen. The best way I can illustrate the value of this frame is by the negative example of one of my patients, Mike.

Mike was planning to go with his wife to a buffet dinner party given by his Aunt Jane, who, according to Mike, made the best German chocolate cake anywhere. He really wanted to have a slice of the cake, but he wanted to do it responsibly, so he worked out the following plan. He would have a slice so thin "you could see light though it"; he would do extra exercise before the party; he would test his blood sugar just before the party and take a little extra insulin to cover the cake; he would cut back on the main course at dinner; and he would test his blood as soon as he came home and take extra insulin if he was high. The plan seemed airtight. The only thing he decided not to do was tell his wife because she was, as he put it, "a real worrywart."

Everything seemed to be going perfectly. When dessert time came my patient even felt his blood sugar was a little low. He could now enjoy his hard-earned treat in all good conscience. As he stood there with his fork poised, about to impale his first mouthful, his wife came charging from across the room, bellowing like a raging bull. "Are you crazy?! Are you trying to kill yourself?" As the man recounted this scene in a session with me several days later, he said the only thing he wanted to do with the cake at that point was smush it in his wife's face. Luckily, he was able to resist this impulse. With the benefit of 20/20 hindsight, he recognized that the disaster was partly his responsibility, since he knew that his wife was a worrier. "I should have bitten the bullet and talked to her beforehand," he said. "I should have told her all that I was doing to make sure I'd be all right, asked her to trust me, and insisted that she stay home if she couldn't, so that she wouldn't ruin my good time."

Positive framing by sharing information starts with the question, What do I need to say and to whom do I need to say it so I can create a mood where something good can happen? This is the question to ask when you're feeling frustrated by how things are going with your health-care provider. If you're not being open about how your diabetes is really going or about how you're feeling, or if you're not satisfied with what you're getting from your provider, you need to find a way to apply the frame of sharing information. This can be hard. Being totally honest or confronting medical authorities often is. But what's the alternative?

The person you need to talk to in order to create the something-good-can-happen mood may be yourself. You may need to consult your Sympathetic Scientist, who's always there waiting in the wings for an honest sharing of information. Only then can the SS help you make good things happen.

THE FRAME OF CELEBRATION

This is the last positive frame, because it's the one that can be used with all the other frames to make them work better. Though I can guarantee that if you can master the skill of positive framing, it will work for you, I can also guarantee that it won't work perfectly all the time, especially at first when you're just getting started. So it's important to develop the habit of celebrating your successes, even when they're small. Perhaps I should say, *especially* when they're small.

Framing positively through celebration begins when you answer the question, How can I celebrate my successes to create an atmosphere in which good things can keep happening? Thomas Edison, himself a diabetic, used this frame to perfection. He had performed 5,000 experiments in his effort to develop the incandescent light bulb without reaching his goal. A reporter interviewed him. "Mr. Edison, how can you continue to pursue this project when you have failed 5,000 times?" Edison looked at the man with a puzzled expression and said, "You say I've failed 5,000 times, but I haven't failed once. I'm just 5,000 steps closer to the ultimate solution." Not too many of us can put such an optimistic twist on our daily experiments with diabetes, but that is the attitude that led to the light bulb and all the rest of Edison's many inventions. Count and celebrate your successes, and they will surely multiply.

June and Barbara: After hearing your explanation about frames, we realize that we've been out there busily reframing the negative into the positive ever since June was first diagnosed. Thank you for giving what we've been doing a name.

Possibly our best achievement in the positive framing area is in the frame of celebrations. June's diabetes was diagnosed on St. Patrick's Day. We remember it well because in those days diabetics tested their urine for sugar and one way to do it was with Tes-Tape, a ribbonlike product that turned a bright Kelly green when the sugar in the urine was really high. Barbara, unconsciously using the frame of humor, suggested to June that she should wear her strip of Tes-Tape in her lapel in honor of the holiday.

At any rate, although many people consider it weird—or even perverse—every year on St. Patrick's Day we celebrate June's diagnosis by doing something wonderful like having an elegant dinner or taking an exciting trip. In 1992—June's twenty-fifth anniversary as a diabetic—we celebrated with a whole Wanderjahr (year of travel) of almost back-to-back trips.

Why do we celebrate? Not because diabetes is such a neat thing to have. We celebrate because, despite diabetes, June is still here, still working, still loving life, still laughing, still doing all the things she wants to do including whatever delightful activity she chooses for her annual celebration.

We believe in the truth of what Shakespeare said in *As You Like It*:

> Sweet are the uses of adversity,
> Which, like the toad, ugly and venomous,
> Wears yet a precious jewel in his head.

Now that we're armed with Dr. Rubin's collection of positive frames, let's all go forth and reframe the toad of diabetes— and all the other toads that may hop into our lives—so that we no longer recoil from their ugliness and fear their venom, but focus instead on the precious jewels they wear in their heads.

The End

INDEX